THE MAGIC IN THE TIN

.

For Bernadette, Elizabeth, Denise, Geraldine, and Isla.
Four brilliant women.
One amazing girl.

THE MAGIC IN THE TIN

A Memoir

PAUL FERRIS

BLOOMSBURY SPORT
LONDON · OXFORD · NEW YORK · NEW DELHI · SYDNEY

BLOOMSBURY SPORT
Bloomsbury Publishing Plc
50 Bedford Square, London, WC1B 3DP, UK
29 Earlsfort Terrace, Dublin 2, Ireland

BLOOMSBURY, BLOOMSBURY SPORT and the Diana logo are trademarks
of Bloomsbury Publishing Plc

First published in Great Britain 2022

A catalogue record for this book is available from the British Library

Library of Congress Cataloguing-in-Publication data has been applied for

ISBN: HB: 978-1-3994-0010-7; eBook: 978-1-3994-0014-5; ePdf: 978-1-3994-0013-8

2 4 6 8 10 9 7 5 3 1

Typeset in Minion Pro by Deanta Global Publishing Services, Chennai, India
Printed and bound in Great Britain by CPI Group (UK) Ltd, Croydon CR0 4YY

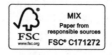

To find out more about our authors and books visit www.bloomsbury.com
and sign up for our newsletters

FOREWORD BY ALAN SHEARER

In November 2017 I wrote the foreword to Paul's first book, *The Boy on the Shed*, and at the end of it I said that he was now a writer as well as a fighter. The accolades and awards the book won were proof of his writing talent.

Nearly five years on, I can repeat that comment – only I may have under-estimated his will to fight.

What Paul has gone through physically, mentally and medically would have knocked many of us over, I firmly believe that. Having had a heart attack, he was then told he had prostate cancer. At the same time, he had a job, he was a dad, a husband, and then a very happy granddad. He had a life to hold together even as he felt his body falling apart.

We all have hurdles put in front of us in life and true resilience is about how you cope. Paul is a shining example that no matter the size of the hurdle, you can still get over it.

He has lost much along the way, as you will read, but not his sense of humour. This is a deeply serious book taking in cancer, surgery, male sexuality, and family, but it is also funny, really funny – I never thought I'd find incontinence so interesting.

Even as a friend of more than 25 years, while I knew Paul was undergoing procedures, I did not know the scale of them. He did not want to tell us, so I wasn't aware of just how raw it all was.

I am now. Paul has spared no detail of what it means for a man to endure prostate cancer and I have no doubt this book will spark a conversation about the grim side effects of treatment and how they can undermine a man's sense of who he is. Paul writes in a revealing, graphic way that few men would dare.

I imagine this book will hit a broader audience than *The Boy on the Shed*. I hope so. It deserves to.

PROLOGUE

In February 2018, something truly remarkable occurred in my life. My memoir, *The Boy on the Shed* was published. That achievement was way beyond my wildest childhood imaginations. My life story to date was met with universal critical acclaim. It led me on an amazing journey. It won multiple awards and was optioned for TV and film. After years of striving and struggle it looked like the shy boy who'd sat on the shed watching over his critically ill mother in the hope she wouldn't leave him was finally destined for great success. My own health troubles, which had resulted in a heart attack in 2013, aged 48, seemed, to anyone who read the book, to be fully behind me.

On the surface all was well in my world. That is how my life appeared. In fact, by the time of publication, my world had already come crashing down around me. A whole other story had emerged between completing the manuscript in 2016 and the publication of my book. Just days after completing my manuscript I'd found myself in a urologist's office hearing the words that none of us want to hear. In the same month I was back in the hospital, this time to welcome my first granddaughter, Isla, into the world. A beacon of light in dark days. A book, prostate cancer and a granddaughter all in the same month. That's the beginning of quite an adventure.

The Magic in the Tin is the story of the journey I have been on ever since. It has taken all of the courage I possess to share some very personal and often humiliating experiences of dealing with the life-changing side effects of my treatments. I hesitated and faltered on numerous occasions before committing to be as honest as I could about the physical and mental challenges I have faced and continue to face. The title itself is a metaphor for having the willingness to embrace life after being dealt some harsh blows. It's true meaning is only revealed in the final paragraphs of the book. Thank you for sharing my story.

Paul Ferris
8 March 2022

CHAPTER 1

It is only autumn still.

I was reflecting on those words as I pulled into the car park in December 2016. They were the ones I'd chosen to finish *The Boy on the Shed,* the memoir I'd been working on since suffering my heart attack in 2013. I'd deliberated long and hard over them. I was pleased with myself that I'd settled on those five words to perfectly encapsulate the frame of mind I was in. I'd had my brush with mortality and winter, but I'd taken decisive action to bulletproof myself against any further heart attacks and the potential catastrophe they would bring to me and my family.

I was looking forward to the hospital appointment. I arrived early. My cardiologist had my blood results from last week. I knew before he smiled at me that they would be good. My year of diet and exercise had guaranteed that.

'Your medication seems to be working well to control your cholesterol. Your blood pressure is optimal, and your weight loss is impressive. You are on target. Just keep doing what you are doing. While I can never say never, I see no reason why you should have another cardiac event Mr Ferris. See you next year.'

Today was a good day. A day to forget the struggles of the past three years and to look forward to the future. I'd done everything I could to ensure my heart disease wouldn't be killing me anytime soon. I'd also just put the finishing touches to my manuscript, which had served to keep me sane and focus my mind through a difficult period in my life. At times I'd felt hopeless and helpless when confronted by the fact that at 48 years of age, I'd not only suffered a heart attack, but that I had an inability to carry cholesterol, which instead of passing through my arteries was sticking to them. The drugs had worked initially. High doses of statins to lower my cholesterol, beta blockers to slow my heart rate, medication to lower my blood pressure, aspirin to thin my blood – the recommended cocktail prescribed to all surviving heart attack patients.

As the weeks and months passed, the side effects of each began to impact on my life to such a degree that there were times when I felt like I could no longer get out of bed. Life as I'd known it with my wife Geraldine, and three boys, Conor, Owen and Ciaran was gone, and gone forever. The thought of that loss had at times robbed me of all hope of any kind of a future. I was the Chief Executive of a growing company, had a great circle of supportive friends and the love of a beautiful family. On the surface, despite the heart attack, I still had so much to look forward to. The sickening reality was very different. As I struggled daily to find my way through my medicated haze, I felt my life was over. All those carefree healthy and happy days I'd taken so much for granted were now firmly in the past. The beta blockers and blood pressure medications ensured I nearly fell over every time I stood up. Light heads and dizzy spells would often force me back into the safety of the chair. While the statins, which I'd initially regarded as miracle drugs because they dramatically lowered my cholesterol, were now becoming my greatest enemy. I felt their hideous effects in my joints at first. I would wince when someone shook my hand or when I turned the handle of a door. Then I felt them in my muscles, which ached with every step I took. I then began to feel so weak that I could no longer pull the quilt over myself at night. I was stuck, locked in this alternative universe, demoralised and defeated. Until one day, at my lowest ebb, I realised that maybe I still had a choice. Yes, I could stay on the medication and live a half-life of dizziness, weakness and pain. Or maybe I could find another way? I chose to try and find the other way.

I read and researched and found my answer in diet and exercise. I could do nothing about the cholesterol my body produced but I didn't have to ingest it as well. So I stopped eating anything that contained cholesterol. I switched my diet overnight dropping all animal products and embarked on a plant-based diet. I didn't find it easy. In fact, I hated it at first. Giving up all my favourite food to focus on eating beans and vegetables felt like an enormous sacrifice, especially as I had never been overly fond of the green stuff. But desperation is a great motivator, and the pains, light heads and dizziness that were wrecking my quality of life were good enough reason to try anything. I increased my exercise and followed my new dietary regime diligently and, like a miracle, I was able to come off almost all of my medications. Within weeks I was down to just a mild dose of statins and an aspirin. I suffered less aches and no pains and was two stone (nearly 13kg) lighter than I was when I'd had my heart attack. More importantly, by the time of my cardiology check-up, I knew my results would be perfect. And the peace of mind that came with knowing that I was doing everything I possibly could to stay fit and well manifested itself in all areas of my life. It was particularly evident in my writing output. I had a manuscript of my life story freshly completed and ready to send off to agents, or publishers, or both. Life was good again. Not as good as before. It never will be. But good enough to look forward to many more years of love and laughter, health and happiness. I was proud to have found the strength to fight for my life and for my family's future. The final sentence of my manuscript perfectly summed up how I felt on that crisp December day.

It is only autumn still.

Those five magic words were still swirling around my head, as I was making my way briskly through the throngs of sick people and heading for the exit of the Royal Victoria Infirmary in Newcastle, when my phone buzzed in my pocket. By the time I'd fumbled for it and nearly dropped it, I was too late to answer it. I looked at the number but didn't recognise it and, because I didn't recognise it, I decided to ignore it. Then the voicemail came through. I listened to the message. It was short and to the point. *The results of your recent biopsy are in. Could you please report to the Freeman Hospital this afternoon to speak with your consultant?* Two separate hospitals in one day. A record even for me with all my recent troubles. I tried to banish all negative thoughts as I slipped my phone into my pocket and started to make my way to my car. I didn't get far. I had intended to, but my legs had different ideas and suddenly lost their ability to carry me there. My dodgy heart was already starting to beat like I was running the 100 metres. Instead of walking I felt for the wall behind me and sat on a tiny ledge jutting from it. I took some deep breaths. Then I did what I always do and what I've always done for the past 37 years when I've received any news, good or bad, in my life; I dialled the most overused number in my address book. Geraldine answered on the first ring.

'How did the appointment go?'

'It was great. Consultant says I'm a star patient. Told me just to keep it up.'

I could hear her sigh on the other end of the line. She had shared every step of the journey with me. The fear, the pain, the hope and the fight.

'Well done. That's brilliant news. You must be relieved. All the hard work has paid off. Anyway, I've got to go. See you later. Love you.'

She was always in a hurry. She teaches in a primary school and the whole world stops while she gives her kids all her time and attention. She'd only answered the phone because she knew about my appointment. Ordinarily she goes 'dark' at school.

'Geraldine, don't hang up!'

There was silence.

'Are you still there?'

'Yes, I'm here. What's up?'

'My biopsy results are in. They want me to go to the Freeman this afternoon to see the consultant. That means only one thing. I think they are going to tell me I have cancer. If that happens, I don't know how I will cope. Not now. After all the efforts I've made with my heart, I can't have cancer as well. Jesus Christ, what is wrong with me? I must have the worst fucking genes in the world. What will I say to the kids? Oh Jesus.'

I didn't hear her at first. She couldn't find a way through my jabbering.

'Paul. Paul! PAUL!'

'What?'

'You don't know anything yet. Let's see what they say first before we panic about anything. I will leave here now and be with you in half an hour. We will go to the hospital together. Whatever the news is we will deal with it. No point in worrying until we have to.'

Her words were sensible, and she was right. I knew nothing. I only knew I'd been asked to go to the hospital for an appointment that afternoon. But that one aspect. Having to report to the hospital on the same day as the results were obtained? To me that was a guarantee that by the time I left that consultation I would be a cancer patient as well as a heart disease patient. The two biggest causes of death in the western world and I would be a sufferer of both. Pretty good going for an ex-professional footballer who'd exercised all my life. I'd only ever smoked one cigarette and that was when my sister Denise had forced me to so I wouldn't tell my mother she smoked like a chimney.

My courage hadn't fully returned before we made our way into the consultant's office. I had long since forgotten my pride at the final sentence of my manuscript. It no longer felt like autumn as I shook his hand and took a seat.

'How are you feeling?'

He had a kind face and gentle manner. I had liked him on my previous consultations with him.

'I'm great. I was the star patient at my cardiology appointment this morning and I've just finished my memoir. So, I'm feeling pretty good.'

I smiled nervously at him. I tried to read his face. Look for some comfort in it. I'd seen him twice before for appointments that had led to the biopsy. He was a straight talker. And I liked that. I could see Geraldine sitting in the chair just behind him. Her calm manner was betrayed by the flushing in her cheeks. He pulled his chair towards me. And delivered the bomb.

'I'm afraid you have prostate cancer. There was a significant amount in both lobes of your gland. I would like you to have a bone scan to rule out the possibility that it has travelled anywhere else in your body. Once that comes back, hopefully clear, then I would recommend we remove your prostate, or you undergo hormone therapy and radiotherapy. No other treatment options are appropriate for you. Because of the volume of cancer and your young age of 51, I think it is highly likely that without treatment, your life will be impacted by this.'

He talked me through my treatment options and the life-changing side effects that seemed to follow any route I chose. I didn't absorb much after he told me I had cancer. I tried to, but my mind was not registering, my ears not hearing. My eyes were working just fine, and I wiped an embarrassing tear away. I shook my head and looked at Geraldine. If the doctor hadn't been sitting between us, I would have raced into her arms. I always felt better there. Nothing frightens me when I'm there. But I wasn't there. I wished I was anywhere else but in that room with the kind doctor telling me I had cancer and blocking my way to Geraldine. But I *was* in that room and he was still speaking. He was speaking but I couldn't hear the words. I could hear something else instead. It started as a whisper at the back of my head and became a roar at the front by the time he'd shaken my confused and dejected hand.

It is only autumn still.

My own words were mocking me. I now had a significant prostate cancer to challenge my heart disease. They could compete with each other. Either one might eventually take me away from everyone and everything I loved, long before my time. How premature I'd been to write those words. I left the room and stepped into Geraldine's arms. She was warm but I was cold. It certainly didn't feel like it was only autumn still. It felt like winter. It felt like nothing would ever be the same. It felt like the beginning of the end.

Every journey must have a start and a finish. I don't yet know how this one ends for me, but I do know where it started. I can take you there. I can take you with me to where it all began. Its origin was eight years ago, in 2014. It commenced with some embarrassment, a fat finger up somewhere it's not meant to go, and some misplaced reassurance.

CHAPTER 2

'Any problems with your waterworks?'

I was getting up to leave when the young doctor spoke to his monitor as it danced off his thick glasses.

I sat back down on the uncomfortable plastic chair.

'No. None. Just the pain in my side.'

The pain in my side was from a troublesome kidney stone I'd been diagnosed with four years previously, in 2010. This appointment was only happening because after my heart attack the previous year, I was determined to get myself into the best shape I possibly could. I'd changed my diet and upped my exercise. I was feeling pretty good, all things considered. Apart from this nagging pain in my side that was my constant companion. I'd been determined to have the stone removed and was not going to take no for an answer this time. That was until the urologist with the dancing glasses explained the procedure he'd recommend to remove the offending stone.

I spent five minutes listening to him tell me all about the process. It would commence with him putting a stent in my penis. He would feed a probe through it and run it all the way up my urethra and into my kidney. He'd pull the stone back along the same route and out through the end of my stented penis. He was very enthusiastic about it all. I had already changed my mind at the 'stent in the penis' part, but out of politeness I let him finish. When he had, my only thought was to get out of his room as quickly as I could. I would never mention my kidney stone again. At least not in the company of someone who had the capability of stenting my penis. I was already on my feet as I was telling him of my change of heart and that the pain in my side was a minor irritation that on reflection, I was more than happy to live with. I declined his invitation to book me in for surgery and apologised for wasting his time. Unfortunately, he wasn't done with me and that's when he asked me the waterworks question. I answered him and told him I had no issues apart from getting up in the night to use the bathroom a little too often.

'Have you had your prostate examined recently Mr Ferris?'

I shuffled in my chair.

'Ah… no. I've not needed to have it checked.'

He already had his glove on and was nodding me towards the bed.

'You're 49 now. I think we should check it while you are here.'

Before I could object, my trousers were down, my knees were tucked up, his finger was up my bum, and he was satisfied. I was mortified. He told me I had an enlarged prostate. It was nothing to worry about. Very common in men of my age. It was firm but not hard, which seemed to mean something to him, but meant nothing to me. I questioned him on it. It should be springy but mine wasn't. Firm and large, nothing to worry about. Hard and lumpy, more of a concern. I left the scene of my violation relieved that I was firm but not hard, smooth but not lumpy.

From that day in 2014, until my diagnosis two years later, I'd never really considered for a moment that I could possibly have prostate cancer. If I'm honest, I didn't really have much of an idea of what my prostate was for anyway. I knew it had something to do with sexual function. Oh… and maybe that some people liked it massaged during the sexual act to heighten the pleasure, but I'd never been inclined to explore that aspect of its purpose myself. I now know this little gland, that sits just below the bladder in men, has an incredibly important role in both sexual and urinary function. It produces the seminal fluid that nourishes and transports semen, plays a role in hormone production, and helps regulate urine flow. In 2014, I was just happy to get out of the room with a firm and smooth one and as far away from the fat finger as I could get.

* * *

It was mid-afternoon in late March 2016, two years after that appointment with the young urologist. I'd just switched the lights on and took a sip of my coffee. My guest was in full flow.

'I was dribbling more than Georgie Best.'

My good friend Peter Hampson was sitting across the boardroom table from me. He would often call in to see me at work and we'd spend an hour or two putting the world to rights. As the years passed, we mostly ended up discussing our mutual failing health. I laughed as he continued to describe the embarrassing troubles he'd been having with his recently diagnosed enlarged prostate. He'd suffered a heart attack and a cardiac arrest six weeks before my own life-changing event.

'Jesus, Peter, we are following the same path to old age. I was diagnosed with that a couple of years back.'

'Really?'

'Yeah. I was having my kidney stone checked a while back and the next thing I know I have a lubricated finger up my bum. Told me I had an enlarged prostate. Said it was firm rather than hard and I shouldn't worry too much about it. Apparently, it's very common in men of a certain age.'

'Old fuckers like us you mean!'

I laughed.

'Unfortunately, I think we are getting to that stage, yes.'

Peter leaned forward in his chair.

'Have you had the piss test, piss flow thing, or whatever it's called? And are you on the tablets as well?'

I shifted uncomfortably in my chair.

'No. Not the tests. Just the diagnosis. You know, the finger up the backside stuff and all that.'

He shook his head.

'If you're dribbling and getting up through the night then you should go back to your doctor and get checked properly. Most of these things are nothing to worry about, but what if it's cancer?'

I suddenly felt uneasy. My symptoms had been getting more noticeable over recent months. I hadn't allowed myself to consider that it could be anything other than an enlarged prostate. I didn't really want to contemplate anything more sinister. I'd had a tough enough time getting to grips with the fact that I'd had a premature heart attack and was now living with a genetic condition that meant I didn't process cholesterol as well as everyone else and was at risk of further heart attacks because of it. One life threatening condition was enough for me for one lifetime. *I couldn't possibly have cancer as well, could I?*

*   *   *

Geraldine switched on her bedside lamp and looked at me with familiar weariness. We'd been talking all evening about my conversation with Peter. I'd just gotten into bed after my third visit to the bathroom since we'd turned in for the night. I'd spent the time in between toilet breaks rambling on about the possibility of having cancer and what that would mean for me, us and our three boys. She sat up and tucked her pillow behind her head to stop the metal frame digging into her.

'I agree with Peter. If you are having symptoms, then you need to go to the doctor. There's no point in worrying about it and talking to me or anyone else. Only the doctor can give you peace of mind. If it is cancer than we will deal with it, just as we have with your heart. Book an appointment tomorrow and we will take it from there.'

I climbed out of bed and made my fourth trek to the bathroom. I lifted the toilet seat and stood in my familiar pose. Nothing came. I gave myself a shake. Still nothing came. I stood a little longer. *For fuck's sake!* I made my way back to the bed. Geraldine switched off her lamp and lay back down. I lay down, then sat back up, flicked on my lamp, got out of bed, and continued what had become my nightly ritual for far too long. A wearily familiar routine I had assumed was caused by my enlarged prostate. I stood in front of the toilet and dribbled into it. One drip, a little dribble, another drip. As I stood exhausted, I tried to remember the last time I'd had a satisfying pee. A year? Maybe two? Longer even? I walked back towards Geraldine, my hand rubbing drips of urine off my thigh. I, too, was now dribbling more than Georgie Best.

'You still awake?'

Geraldine turned around and shielded her eyes from the lamplight (or maybe my middle-aged body).

'Of course I'm not asleep, with you up and going to the toilet every five minutes.'

I climbed in beside her and she laid her head on my chest.

'This obviously isn't right. Up and down all night and going more when I'm on my way back than I do when I'm there. I need to get it sorted one way or another. I'll call the doctor tomorrow.'

She breathed heavily on my chest. I thought about asking her to move so I could go back to the toilet. I let her sleep instead and trudged back to the bathroom as soon as she turned around and settled down for the night. When I returned, I lay in the darkness and let my fears wash over me. I thought about our three boys asleep in their rooms; of how life turns so quickly; of how solid and how certain everything had seemed before my heart attack; of the illusion of invincibility we build around ourselves and our lives. It can all unravel so quickly, sometimes without warning. Sometimes it can unravel slowly too, with an extra dribble at the end of a toilet visit, or a slight delay before the act itself begins. I tried not to think about anything other than calling the doctor in the morning. Instead, I thought about nothing else other than what would happen to Geraldine and the boys if I had cancer, if I couldn't work, if I was gone.

Geraldine stirred, and pulled the quilt off me as she did every night. A drowsy tug of war usually followed, but not tonight. Tonight, she could have her victory. I leaned across, kissed her back, told her I loved her, and slid once more out of the bed. After my latest failed attempt to deposit anything meaningful into the toilet, I opened the bedroom door and crept downstairs in the darkness, ignoring my natural reticence to do so. Since childhood I've been afraid of the dark and ordinarily would switch on every light in the house, just in case something dreadful jumped out and attacked me before I'd made it from the bedroom to the kitchen.

The kettle sprung noisily into life as I stared at my reflection in the kitchen window. My ghost looked back at me, pale, gaunt, haunted.

My trance was broken by movement outside in the darkness. I yelped, jumped back, and was glad no one was there to witness my latest act of bravery. I didn't look out of the window again as I poured the hot water into my cup.

I sat at the kitchen table and pushed my laptop to the side to rest my cup in front of me. The laptop was only on the table, as earlier, I'd been putting the finishing touches to the latest chapter of the memoir I'd been writing. It was originally entitled *So You Did* – three little words that had meant so much to me as a young boy growing up in Ireland. My football coaches at Lisburn Youth would shout them every time I scored my latest goal or pulled off my latest trick. Their confidence in me, when I had none in myself, had ensured I progressed all the way to becoming a professional footballer and the youngest player ever to play for Newcastle United. That's what the memoir was about – my journey from Ireland – leaving everything I loved behind, including my ill mother, Bernadette, and my girlfriend, Geraldine. It had been quite a rollercoaster and had culminated in my unexpected heart attack in 2013. I'd spent the last three years physically and mentally fighting my way back and was finally making great progress with both.

So You Did would eventually become *The Boy on the Shed*. The new title would be a direct reference to me sitting on an old coal bunker outside our home in Ireland. I'd climb up there every day after my mother had suffered the first of her many heart attacks. I'd peer at her though the kitchen window and believed that if I was watching over her then she wouldn't leave me. Her first heart attack had occurred while I was sleeping, oblivious beside her. I was five years old. I'd like to claim credit for the eventual title, but it had nothing to do with me. It would come from a moment of inspiration from elsewhere.

I wasn't ready to go back to bed. I knew my racing brain wouldn't settle in the darkness of the bedroom. I opened the laptop and scrolled down to the last chapter I'd written earlier. I sat and stared at the blank space below. I began to type… and type… and type. When I closed the laptop, I had a further two chapters written. It was daylight when I stood up to put my empty cup in the sink. I stared out of the window. Light was streaming into the courtyard. The branches of a tree were swaying backwards and forwards. The scary monsters of the night-time were nothing to be frightened of in the bright morning light.

I crawled into bed beside Geraldine and pressed my cold body against her warm one. She curled up and pulled the quilt around her. The last few years, suffering the heart attack and now the fear that I might have cancer as well, had obliterated almost all of the certainty that was in my life. But as I played tug of war with my sleeping wife, I still had one constant that I knew I could rely on. My quilt thief would stand by my side whatever the future held for me. I gave up the fight again and let her steal it away. I kissed her warm back, whispered to it that I was frightened, and told it I loved it. Then I got up and dripped and dribbled into the toilet once more before birdsong finally rocked me to sleep. I needed to phone the doctor first thing in the morning. No matter how uncomfortable that thought made me feel.

CHAPTER 3

The bloody internet!

In the two days between making my appointment at the doctors and trudging my way into the characterless building that houses my GP, I had convinced myself 10 times that I was suffering from an enlarged prostate, 20 times that I did in fact have prostate cancer and 30 times I was going to be dead within the year. No matter how many times I told myself not to search for my symptoms, I'd find myself staring into my phone late into the night as Geraldine hogged the quilt beside me.

Not only that, but I knew exactly what was in store for me during the examination. I was very relieved when I was called into the room by a gentleman I didn't recognise rather than Dr Green, my usual GP. If someone was going to slip a finger up my backside I would rather it was a stranger. That doesn't sound right does it? For clarity, I'm not suggesting I like a stranger sticking a finger up my bum, but if I had to have a digit up there then I don't want it to belong to someone I'm familiar with. That doesn't sound any better, I know. The locum GP didn't bother with any small talk and got straight to it.

'Any family history of prostate cancer?'

I'd barely sat my nervous bum on the chair and mentioned the Georgie Best dribbling and he was on the cancer questions right away. I tried to put him off the scent.

'Yes, my brother Joseph has prostate cancer, but he has heart disease and has had a bypass. I think he has diabetes and Crohn's disease too. He has everything. My other brothers are OK, and my father was fine. Apart from when he died. Obviously, he wasn't fine that day. But it wasn't prostate cancer that killed him. He never had a problem in that department and neither have I.'

I was on a roll now.

'I've already been examined by a urologist a couple of years back and he did a digital rectal examination and was happy that my delay in micturition was due to the enlarged prostate he palpated. Firm but not hard, smooth not lumpy, and the sulcus was intact. My symptoms have worsened a little, but they are not too bad.'

That was him told. He now knew I knew my stuff alright. Family history nonsense firmly put in its place. He was totally unmoved by my internet-based knowledge. He spoke while fingering his keyboard. A precursor of things to come.

'I'd like to palpate your prostate if I may? It may feel a little uncomfortable, but I will be very brief.'

I shifted in my chair. The thought of a second finger up my backside caused a bead of sweat to trickle down my forehead and my about-to-be-parted buttocks to clench tightly.

'Is that really necessary?'

He was already up, gloved, and walking towards the treatment table which occupied about a third of the floor space in his cramped office.

'I'm afraid so. Could you climb on the bed, lower your trousers, turn on your side and raise your knees to your chest for me?'

I could, but I'd rather not.

I did what I was told. Defeated, I plodded towards the table. He pulled a curtain while I climbed onto the bed and undid my jeans and slid them to my knees. I turned on my side to face the wall and focused on a small hole in the plaster that needed filling in. Ten seconds later, his absurdly thick finger was forcing its way up my freshly lubricated back passage. What is it with doctors and fat fingers? The other fella's wasn't too thin either. They should measure finger girth as part of the entry requirements for getting into medical school. Too fat and you're not getting on the course. Never mind your great education and four A*s. *Fuck off and do law instead and spare middle-aged men's bottoms from unnecessary trauma, stumpy.*

For the period a finger is up your bottom and poking at your prostate it feels like having a big poo backwards. Very unpleasant. It might be my Irish Catholic upbringing, but I can't for the life of me imagine being in the throes of passion with another human being and she just slips a finger up my bum and rummages around to find my prostate to massage. One minute it's all Marvin Gaye and sweet nothings and then the next her finger is up my bum. It would give a whole new meaning to Marvin's *What's Going On*. No matter how much in love we were, or how well we knew each other, that would be the end of the relationship right there. A finger up my bum without asking permission? No thank you. Come to think of it, someone asking permission is even worse. Unless she was a doctor... and I wasn't having sex with that doctor at the time the question was asked.

My latest violation was more unpleasant than the last one. He seemed to do a lot more rummaging, and his finger was definitely fatter than my previous intruder's. Thankfully, it was over quickly. I was soon seated on my freshly assaulted behind and listening to the softly spoken doctor as he explained his 'concerns' to me.

'Your prostate is smooth, which is good news. But it feels hard rather than springy. I also can't find a distinct sulcus, which makes me a little uneasy about leaving you without further tests.'

My late-night internet searches had informed me that 'hard' and 'no sulcus' wasn't good.

'Your prostate does feel a little enlarged though.'

That was better. It was just as the other doctor had surmised. The internet said that was good. Maybe it was a benign enlarged prostate after all? He could stick his finger up my bum anytime if that was going to be his diagnosis. An appointment for Peter's piss test, some medication and let's forget the whole thing. Nothing to see here. Move on. But he wasn't finished.

'However, it doesn't feel particularly large to me.'

Bugger!

'I'd like to do a PSA test. For a man of your age, the amount of prostate-specific antigen in your blood should be at a certain level. If we do the test, coupled with the examination we've just had, then it will give us a much better idea of just what we are looking at. If the results are elevated, then that is a sign that you are having some issues with your prostate.'

I'd read all about PSA tests. *Not accurate, can't determine if elevated results are from an enlarged prostate or a cancerous one, can give false negative and false positive results.* That was just the view from the medical experts. The input from the great unwashed on the internet was that a PSA test would lead me to an unnecessary biopsy, a risk of infection and lots of other outcomes that I hadn't even allowed myself to contemplate. Then there were the loud and proud brigade, who informed me that I shouldn't ever have any investigations because even if it was prostate cancer, it would be so slow growing that it would likely never amount to anything significant enough to trouble me. Therefore, I'd be mad to put myself through all the physical and mental trauma that would follow a diagnosis of prostate cancer. I was still smarting from the fat finger.

'Do I really need to have the PSA test? A urologist and you have both performed rectal examinations and found my prostate to be enlarged. Surely that is the most likely cause of my symptoms?'

He crossed his legs, locked his chubby fingers together, and placed them on his knee.

'It may well be that your enlarged prostate is causing your urinary symptoms, however, I have some concerns after my examination and I really think you should have a PSA test. I have to point out that once you have it, then it may lead you down a further path, with more investigations to get to the bottom of everything.'

I looked up and smiled at the last line. He stared blankly back at me, all doctorly, offending finger locked around the others. Not even a 'pardon the pun'. We stared at each other in silence, I thought about putting up some further internet-based arguments as to why he, as a doctor, was entirely wrong, and why Brad, from Massachusetts, and Gunter from Dusseldorf knew better. I decided the best course of action was to agree with him and buy myself some time.

'If you think I should have the test then I will. When do you want me to come back to see the nurse?'

I just wanted to get out of the room and thought my agreement to come back and see the nurse would do the job. When I was safely out of there, I would then have time to gather my thoughts properly. I could go home and speak to Geraldine. Spend several hours on the internet. Or do nothing. Just forget about the whole thing and dribble my way into old age like thousands of men before me, before PSA tests and the other advances in medicine. It didn't do my father's generation any harm. Come to think of it, he did spend a long time at the urinal in the pub and he definitely dribbled a lot. I thought that was just a by-product of copious pints of Guinness. Maybe he had undiagnosed prostate cancer? That would mean two members of my immediate family with it. Maybe my other brothers had it too and just didn't know it yet? With our genes that would be highly likely. We'd been to a family wedding recently and I'd shared a table with two of my brothers and my two sisters. I'd gone around the table and jokingly identified them all by their ailments. There were far too many for people of our age. Most were cardiovascular, the odd heart attack here and there, bypasses and stents, some surgery to unblock a carotid artery, a sprinkling of diabetes, and a touch of Crohn's disease – but no cancer. We'd laughed at the hopelessness of the genetic hand we'd all been dealt. Maybe cancer lurked there too, and we just didn't know? I owed it to myself and my family to get checked properly. No procrastinating. Just get the test done. The doctor interrupted my cataloguing of familial diseases and made my mind up for me.

'Just roll your sleeve up and I will do it now for you.'

He was far too keen and annoyingly efficient, but he was right. I offered him my best vein. With my PSA test done and on its way to the lab, I exited the surgery and made my way to the car. In the three years since we'd moved into our new home and I'd registered with this new GP practice, I'd had a heart attack and was now being tested for prostate cancer. In the 15 years at my previous surgery, I don't think I visited it more than three times. Some two years on from my heart attack I had completely overhauled my lifestyle. I'd only done that out of desperation to get rid of my joint and muscle pain, but I was glad I had. The debilitating pains had set me off on a quest to find a way to get off my statins and get some quality of life back.

To my great relief, the more I had read around the subject of diet, the more evidence I'd found from very eminent doctors, that heart disease didn't have to be a slow inevitable decline into ever-clogging arteries and an early grave. I may well have stumbled upon it through desperation, but I'd grasped the opportunity to fight against the path my genes had laid out for me, and I was convinced I was winning the battle. I was only taking a very mild dose of statins (5 milligrams, 3 days a week, compared to 80 milligrams every day previously), and yet my cholesterol levels had dropped to the lowest levels they'd ever been in my entire life. All my aches and pains had subsided. It had felt like a miracle. My mind had cleared of the fog that had descended after the heart attack and I had even started writing my memoir. I didn't truly believe it would ever be published, but writing it filled my evenings with pleasure and helped me move on from the dark days after my heart attack. I was also back in good spirits at work and very much looking forward to the future. Now this prostate issue had come along. Just because of a few dribbles of piss, my head was filling with worry and angst once again. Surely I couldn't have had an early heart attack, and now have cancer at 51? It felt particularly cruel.

I closed the car door and started the engine. The car radio sparked into life and I smiled to myself. Marvin Gaye serenaded me with *What's Going On*. I drove the short distance from the GP's thick finger to the supermarket to buy vegetables for my meatless, and most likely, tasteless dinner. Trying to stay alive was literally becoming a pain in the arse.

CHAPTER 4

Life goes on as normal when you are waiting for test results that might change it forever. Everything is normal until it no longer is. It was April 2016. My eldest son, Conor and his girlfriend, Kayleigh, had just surprised us with the news that we were to be grandparents. I didn't know then just how important that new arrival in my life would become for my mental well-being in the months and years that followed. Conor would soon be looking for a place to live with his young family. Our middle son, Owen, was coming to the end of his time in high school and we were dreading the day he would leave home and make his way to university, like thousands of other excited teenagers. Ciaran, our baby, wasn't a baby anymore, and had started his GCSE studies. We would soon be transitioning from a full house to a practically empty one.

We live in a beautiful barn conversion in the hills outside of the town of Prudhoe, in Northumberland. We'd moved here in 2011, after living in an equally beautiful, rented home in the village of Heddon-on-the-Wall. Both moves followed the almighty mess I'd gotten us into by flirting with a career in professional football management. I'd jumped off a more secure pathway as a barrister to accompany Alan Shearer into what I thought would be a long and distinguished career in football management. The failure of that to materialise had finally ended my long association with professional football, and Newcastle United in particular. I'd spent 18 years of my life at the club, first as a player, then as a physiotherapist and, all too briefly, as head of the medical department during Alan's short tenure as manager in 2009. That adventure, which began at home in Ireland, featured many twists and turns and ended in the present day. It also occupied my every evening, providing the rich material for *The Boy on the Shed*. It usually had me tapping furiously into my laptop while Geraldine sat opposite me at the kitchen table, working through the never-ending paperwork she brought home from school every night.

'Are your two fingers broken?'

I looked up from the blank screen. Geraldine was peering over her glasses and her laptop.

'What?'

She lifted a glass of wine to her lips and sat it back down. It balanced precariously on the lead of her own laptop before she guided it to the safety of the kitchen table. Our dog Ollie heard the noise. He lifted his head from its resting place at my feet. He had a quick look to see if any food was on offer, before he slumped back down and exhaled loudly.

'Your two fingers. You are usually typing at least 10 words a minute with them by this stage. You've been sitting there for an hour and haven't typed a thing.'

I picked her wine glass up and brought it to my nose. I inhaled and then put my lips to the glass. I licked the bitter wine with my tongue and thought about sharing a glass with her for the first time since I'd stopped drinking just after Christmas. Instead, I handed it back to her and stood up to boil the kettle.

'What's the point of all the dietary stuff, no drinking, and exercising, if I'm going to have cancer now too?'

She got up and walked behind me. She spun me around and hugged me tightly.

'We don't know anything yet, but I do know that you looking after yourself has been the best thing you have done for yourself, and all of us, since your heart attack. It is good for the kids to see you making an effort and not just giving up on everything. It would be really stupid to undo all the good work because you are a bit stressed about some test results that might turn out to be fine anyway.'

I let go and reached for a cup. I was going to protest that she had a glass of wine on the table and had just eaten a ribeye steak an hour ago, while I'd had a black bean burger and some water, but I resisted. I knew she was right. I could have eaten what she had but my body wouldn't have processed it like hers did. She could have her steak and wine. I'd made the decision to fight my genes and I would continue to do so. I owed that to her and to my boys. But tonight, the manuscript would have to wait. The only thing on my mind were the results of the PSA test and what they would mean for my future.

I got them quite quickly. My mobile rang while I was in a board meeting at work. I'd formed a company, Speedflex, with hugely successful businessman Graham Wylie and Alan Shearer in 2011. We'd created a small-group high-intensity interval-training concept, and we'd successfully sold dedicated Speedflex studio equipment into several gyms across the UK and Ireland. The three of us were in full flow on our latest set of challenges when I had to excuse myself and step out of the room. I'd recognised the GP practice number and had to take the call. It had only been two days since my examination and blood test.

'Is that Mr Ferris?'

I recognised Dr Green's voice.

'Dr Green. Good afternoon.'

He got straight to the point as always.

'We've had the results back from your recent PSA test and I'm afraid the readings are quite high for a man of your age. Your reading is 9.3 and I would expect a man of your age to be around 1, certainly no more than 3. I wouldn't be happy leaving matters like this, and I would like to refer you to a urologist who may very well choose to do a biopsy and some further tests. I...'

I interrupted his flow with my 'Brad from Massachusetts' argument.

'I've read you can get false positive results, and that certain labs give different results. Could there be a mistake?'

He sighed down the line.

'There can sometimes be false positives and negatives. Like if you had recently ejaculated or ridden a bicycle. That can elevate the reading somewhat. I ...'

'I have!'

'What?'

'Ridden a bicycle and ejaculated before the test.'

Not at the same time as that would be a bit weird. He sighed again. Like he didn't believe me. He was right not to believe me. I'd done neither.

'In that case, could we book you an appointment for a repeat test as soon as possible?'

There was a short pause.

'And if you could refrain from riding a bike and ejaculating just prior to it, then I'm sure we will get an accurate reading.'

I didn't really care that the doctor now suspected I was a liar. Or worse that he now thought I rode around the north east of England masturbating on my bike. Or even worse still, he suspected that the excitement of the ride was such that it caused me to spontaneously erupt over the handlebars. I just wanted another test. I simply couldn't believe that my PSA was 9.3. If it was 9.3, I knew what that meant. The higher the PSA, the more likely it was cancer, rather than an enlarged prostate. There was a bell curve of probability and I was on the wrong side of it. I went back to my meeting, cheeks flushed and head spinning. The boss of a health and fitness company with heart disease and now cancer maybe? I wished I *had* been masturbating on a bike. At least I would have had some hope that the next test result would be different. The next test result was different. It was worse.

'Your PSA has come back at 9.4.'

It was Dr Green again. He had a very nice manner and delivered the bad news gently. I had nowhere else to go. No bikes. No ejaculations. No nothing. Just the knowledge that I had a very elevated PSA and there was a distinct possibility that I had prostate cancer.

'What happens next then?'

'You will receive a letter from the hospital and should have an appointment with a urologist shortly after that. I'm sorry, I know this is a very uncertain time but I'm not happy just leaving matters as they are, what with your family history and now two test results on the high side.'

He was right about the letter. I got one within a week, telling me where I had to go and who I was to see there. It made everything seem so urgent. Like maybe I was on some 'fast track to diagnosis' protocol. It unnerved me a little how quickly things were moving. But I was also happy that the uncertainty would soon be over. I'd know very soon whether or not I had prostate cancer, what stage it was at, what treatment I would get, and what the whole thing meant for my prospects of hanging around for a few more years. I was mentally prepared for whatever was to come at the hastily arranged urologist appointment. That was until I got another letter telling me to ignore the previous letter and that I would get a further letter telling me where I had to go and the name of the other urology team member who would be more suitable for me to consult with. I was quite encouraged by that letter. I guessed that if they were cancelling the first one within two weeks and were now telling me to wait for another letter some unspecified time in the future, that that could only mean one thing. My situation wasn't so urgent after all. Some other poor people needed the two-week follow-up protocol. The less urgent people like me, who were unlikely to have cancer after all and who were more likely to just have an enlarged prostate, could wait their turn. I was happy to wait my turn.

I was glad to forget about the whole thing until I needed to think about it again. I put it to the back of my mind. No searching the internet, or boring Geraldine with my woes, no PSA chats, no prostate chats and certainly no cancer conversations. In fact, I didn't give the letters and upcoming rearranged appointment any thought at all. If anything, I would go as far as to say I forgot all about it. The trouble is, so did they... whoever *they* were. One minute it was all urgent PSA tests, repeat PSA tests, urgent letters and two-week timeframes, and the next, I'm getting on with my days and dribbling my way through my nights, working and writing, dribbling and wiping.

Months passed with no contact from the hospital. Work was going well. I was making great progress writing *The Boy on the Shed*, and my vegan diet and my daily sessions on Speedflex had helped me shed 35lb (19kg) in weight. We set off at the end of July 2016 on a dream holiday to Boston, Cape Cod and New York. It would most likely be the last holiday our family would have together before Conor moved out, and Owen moved on too. The holiday was everything I hoped it would be. I loved the culture and the Irish feel of Boston and was very much looking forward to five days in New York. While we were in Cape Cod, we took advantage of the fact that Coldplay were performing at Patriots Stadium in Foxborough. Halfway through the performance, I looked along the row to my left. Geraldine was cheering, Conor and Owen were sharing a joke and a beer, and Ciaran stood wide-eyed and engrossed in the moment. And it was a moment. Just a fleeting moment, but my eyes filled with tears of gratitude and pride in the family I shared my life with. Life was good again. I was content. Then everything came to a shuddering halt.

I had entered the gents with Ciaran and a steady stream of excited Americans, during a brief lull in the concert. I slipped into a spot that had been vacated by a swaying drunk in a beer-stained Boston Celtics top. I unbuttoned my jeans, prepared to dribble my way into the metal trough and waited. The man next to me was peeing like a shire horse. So much so that I could feel splashes of his impressive efforts bouncing onto my hands and jeans. He left and was replaced by an equally forceful pisser. He too left and the next performer staggered into me before matching, maybe even eclipsing, the performance of his predecessors. I looked down into the bowl in front of me. The strong-smelling disinfectant tablet, that acted as my target, remained bone dry. I shook my useless hose again. I felt like I was ready to go, any minute now there would be a trickle, a weak flow, a dribble and another dribble. But this time nothing came.

'Hey buddy, are you gonna move along, or stand there with your dick in your hand all night? I'm missing the show, man.'

I turned to tell the deep voice to fuck off and mind his own business. My head came face to face with his muscular chest. I looked up and decided to let him have his moment. I buttoned my jeans and made my way out through the one-way system and back into the concourse. I hadn't spilled a drop. Not one solitary drip of urine. I felt nauseous as I approached Ciaran who was waiting patiently. He turned to walk back to our seats but I got back in the queue for the gents again. Coldplay were no doubt on brilliant form on that hot night in the summer of 2016. I could tell they were by the reaction of the excited fans, and the looks on the faces of those I loved most in the world. But as for myself, I can't remember if they were good, bad or indifferent. I spent the rest of the concert cursing myself and my genes. *So, I couldn't even piss now?* That's not technically true. By the second visit to the toilet, I was back to dripping and dribbling. But the first one had terrified me. I sweated and fretted my way through the remainder of the show. How had I not been able to piss? What was stopping me? An enlarged prostate or cancerous one? Why were my symptoms getting worse? Was the cancer I may not even have growing, spreading, blocking… and why the fuck had the hospital not sent me a letter with an appointment date on it?

CHAPTER 5

It became clear pretty quickly why I hadn't received my letter or new appointment at the hospital. After much procrastination on my part and some exasperation on Geraldine's, I called the number on the original letter. I needn't have bothered.

'You're through to the wrong place. We just send the letters out. I can't help you and I don't know why you haven't received a follow-up letter. They are issued through your doctor or your local hospital. I suggest you call them.'

Her tone was cold and aloof. I wanted to shout down the phone that I was a patient trying to establish whether or not I had cancer. Couldn't she show a little more understanding, patience, humanity even? Instead, I hung up and made several more calls. Finally, I got through to a secretary to one of the urologists at the Freeman Hospital in Newcastle. She was very apologetic and much more helpful.

'You have slipped off the system. I don't know why that is, but please accept my apology. I will get a new appointment date sent out to you as soon as possible. Apologies again.'

So that was it. Somewhere between my urgent two-week appointment and the cancellation of it, I had slipped through the system. My PSA test had been done (twice) in April. It was now October. All the while I was busy enjoying myself at work, at home, and on holiday, safe in the knowledge that if there was any urgency around my blood tests that the hospital would have contacted me. The simple fact was that I, and my potential prostate cancer, had disappeared off the radar. I felt my cheeks flush and my palms moisten at the thought of it. Six months had passed since my concerned GP with the stumpy finger had thought my results merited an urgent follow up. *Six months! Fuck!*

I may well have slipped off the system but that didn't mean that whatever was stopping me pissing and making me miss too much of a Coldplay concert had disappeared. My symptoms hadn't vanished. In fact, if anything, they'd gotten worse. It was at night I noticed the changes the most. My sleep was interrupted so much that I would wake in the morning and feel as tired as I had when I had climbed into bed the night before. Even during the day, my lack of ability to have a satisfactory pee was getting more and more frustrating for me. But mostly I tried to put it to the back of my mind and get on with my work and my life. Now, knowing I should have been seen after two weeks but instead had been drifting for months, ensured my mind was racing. If it was cancer, then it had just had another six months to grow and multiply and attack my body. Wasn't early diagnosis the key to beating cancer? I could feel the anger building. How could I be allowed to float around the place thinking everything was fine, when in fact I'd just fallen through the cracks? Surely my life and my family's future were worth more than that? I cursed myself for not being more forceful. When the second letter hadn't come, I should have been straight on the phone. And it shouldn't have to be that difficult for a patient to get an appointment to establish whether or not they have a life-threatening disease growing inside them. It was 2016, not 1816.

I carried my anger around with me for the next few days. I shared it with my family and work colleagues, snapping at Geraldine and the boys, disengaging from my responsibilities at work. Every time I saw an advert on the TV about the great strides we were all making in defeating cancer, and the importance of research and early diagnosis in that fight, it just made me sick to the pit of my stomach. Any website I browsed regarding diagnosis and treatment for prostate cancer, delivered the same message. Prostate cancer was only a killer if the patient left it too late to report symptoms to a doctor. Early diagnosis was the key to survival. A six-month lag between my initial contact with my GP and a follow up with a consultant seemed unacceptable. It would have been a lot longer, or maybe never, had I not called again. The thought of this destructive thing that might be growing inside me made me shudder every time I let it enter my head. Mostly though, I still lived in hope that it was a benign enlarged prostate. It was more than hope I think. In my calmer, more rational moments, that is what I *believed* it was. I had cause for optimism. After all, most of the websites I read told me that an enlarged prostate was the most likely cause of my symptoms and that cancer was far less likely in a man of my age. I just needed to know one way or the other. I checked the post daily, in the hope that my letter of appointment was there.

As it happened, I didn't have to wait long at all for my six-months-late appointment. Before I knew it, I was slipping out of my office in Jesmond, and sitting in a sterile reception area at the urology clinic at the Freeman Hospital in Gosforth. Geraldine had offered to come with me, but I'd dismissed her attempt at support as being an over-the-top response to a follow-up appointment I should have had months before. Nothing much would happen apart from another finger up my bum. I didn't need her, or anybody there to witness that. Not inviting her to the initial appointment was my attempt to deny the possible seriousness of the situation.

I waited in the holding pen for over an hour as the sick people were called, one by one, to find out how far their cancers had spread, or regressed, since they had last sat in the crowded waiting area. Or maybe they weren't so sick and were all just disappearing through a door and pissing up a wall, before getting their medication for their 'nothing to worry about' benign enlarged prostates.

'Mr Ferris please.'

I'd been playing with my phone and didn't hear the nurse's voice over the murmuring of the ailing, or not so ailing, masses. I felt a tap on my shoulder. I looked up to see a familiar face in an unfamiliar environment.

'I thought it was your name when I saw the notes in the office this morning. Come with me. The doctor is ready for you now.'

Her name was Julie Needham. I knew her as a longstanding member of Speedflex. She'd been someone who'd always had a ready smile and a kind demeanour. She was the senior nurse in the urology department. She spent her days comforting and consoling cancer patients or telling the not-so-sick ones how to take their medications to ease the frequency of their nightly visits to the toilet and embarrassing dribbling. She led me down a crowded hallway filled with uniforms, suits and stethoscopes, and cluttered with trolleys bursting with bulging notes. She opened the third door on the right and introduced me to Mr Jonathan Alderton. He smiled warmly, shook my hand firmly, and ushered me into an empty chair at the end of his desk. He sat facing me and side-on from his computer screen, which he stared at intensely. Julie perched on the treatment couch behind him. He didn't look up from the screen as he began to speak softly.

'Before we continue, Mr Ferris, I understand that Julie is known to you. If you would rather she wasn't here for our consultation, then she will leave the room.'

I suddenly felt very uncomfortable. *Why would she need to leave the room for a follow-up appointment of a GP referral made six months ago?* I looked nervously over his shoulder towards Julie, who was leaning forward, sitting on her hands, and getting ready to leave.

'No, that's fine. I'm happy for her to stay.' *Why wouldn't I be? Nothing to see here.*

He continued to scrutinise his computer screen as he spoke.

'How are you feeling? Are you generally well? No aches and pains?'

'Apart from the heart attack, stent, heart disease, and statin aches, I'm doing pretty well.'

I thought my response might lighten the mood in the room a little. It didn't.

'Do you have any siblings who suffer from prostate cancer?'

He turned his head to face me.

'Yes. My brother, Joseph, has it.'

He nodded his head knowingly.

'I see and how…'

I didn't let him finish. I'd read the literature too.

'Yes, but he also has Crohn's disease, diabetes, heart disease and goodness knows what else. My other three brothers are all fine, as was my father.'

He looked at the screen and then back at me.

'I think you have a significant cancer.'

He waited for me to answer. I didn't disappoint. I could feel the anger rush through me.

'You're joking right?'

His face and his tone suggested otherwise.

'You've had two PSA test results of 9.3 and 9.4, and you have a brother with prostate cancer. If I enter those details into the algorithm, there is a 40% chance you have the disease. Given your age and your symptoms, I think the likelihood is that you have a significant cancer. By that, I mean one that will impact on your life if we don't intervene.'

I could hear him, but I was no longer listening. *A significant cancer?* Just like that. No tests. No fat finger up the bum. Just a doctor looking at test results I'd had six months previously. *That couldn't be right, surely?*

'I don't understand. Those results have been there for months. For six months, I've been wandering around the north east thinking everything was fine. It was me that had to call your department to get this appointment. Yet now without any further tests, or you knowing for sure whether I even have cancer or not, you've just told me you think I have a significant cancer? That can't be right.'

He dismissed my protest.

'I don't think the six months will make much of a difference. Prostate cancer is a slow growing cancer. I would like to do an MRI scan to check the surrounding areas, and then follow that up with a special type of biopsy. This will be done under general anaesthetic, and it will make sure we get an accurate diagnosis.'

Maybe it was the shock at the sudden bluntness of his manner, or fear, or the fact that I'd done altogether too much internet searching, but whatever it was, I was now in the mood for an argument.

'Couldn't it still be an enlarged prostate? The PSA test is notoriously inaccurate and leads to unnecessary biopsies. Don't the biopsies themselves sometimes lead to infections and the spread of cancer cells outside the prostate? What will happen to me if I choose to walk out of here and forget this entire conversation? You just said prostate cancer was slow growing. Maybe it will never impact on my life. That's if I even have it in the first place.'

That was all I could think of in the short time I'd had to construct my argument. I was happy with the objections I'd raised. He obviously wasn't. He sighed and rocked back in his chair. His tone hardened.

'If you walk out of that door, Mr Ferris, I will put a huge red line through your notes, and I will write a further note to say you have ignored medical advice. I've spoken to lots of men in your situation. Don't be someone who comes back into the system years down the line when it is too late for us to help you. Right now, you are a young man with your life ahead of you. If you were 81, and we were having this conversation, then I might agree with some of what you've just said, but you are not 81, you are 51, and I think you might have a significant cancer. The only way to find out for sure is to have the MRI, and depending on what we find from that, possibly a biopsy to follow.'

By the time he had finished speaking, my anger had subsided and had been replaced by resignation. I admired his professionalism and he certainly had the confident air of someone who knew he was good at his job. I would rather have been anywhere else but in his consulting room, but if I had to be in one, I was comfortable that this was the right one... albeit six months late. I shook his hand and conceded the argument.

My legs were a little unsteady as I made my way from his room. Julie ushered me into an empty consultation room opposite. I turned to face her as she followed me into the cluttered space. She reached out her arms and hugged me. I could feel a tear build in the corner of my eye. I pulled away and wiped it all in one movement, in the hope that she hadn't noticed.

'Why didn't you speak with me when I was at Speedflex, Paul?'

I hadn't spoken with her, because while I knew she was a nurse, I hadn't known she was a urology nurse who dealt with cancer patients. I certainly never expected that I'd be seeing her in any sort of professional capacity. She had a calming nature, and I left the room in a better state than I'd entered it. By the time I got home and waited for Geraldine, I'd managed to rationalise my conversations with the doctor. It wasn't great that I might have prostate cancer, and a significant one at that. But then that wasn't what he'd said exactly. He'd said there was a 40 per cent chance I had a significant cancer. That was still a 60 per cent chance that I didn't. He'd also reluctantly conceded that I may not have cancer at all and that was why I needed the further tests. That didn't sound too bad in my head. When I tried to relay the day's events to Geraldine, I attempted to put a positive spin on it. My eyes didn't agree with my reasoning. I gave up and sobbed on her shoulder instead.

CHAPTER 6

The Boy on the Shed, or should I say, *So You Did,* kept me sane. The manuscript I'd been working on since my heart attack was almost complete. As I sat down to write the latest chapter of my memoir, I felt a pang of loss for happy, fun-filled days, long since passed. Where had they gone? When did they go? Were they ever coming back? I knew the answers to where they'd gone and when. Leaving home in Ireland at 16 to become a professional footballer at Newcastle United had taken care of most of it. My unexpected heart attack had sorted out the rest. Sitting there at the kitchen table in front of the blank screen of my laptop, I felt like they were never coming back. I'd fought so hard to get as healthy as I could after my heart attack, yet here I was dribbling my way from the toilet to the kitchen table and back again while trying to write an uplifting ending to my memoir.

I looked across the table at Geraldine, busily typing her never-ending workload into her own laptop. She peered over her glasses at the screen. I was never sure why she wore them, if they were just an obstacle to be overcome. I felt a knot in my stomach when I looked at her. All of our hopes, all of our dreams, all of our plans, some of which we'd been making since I met her when she was a 13-year-old girl and I was a 15-year-old boy back in Lisburn, had all turned to dust with my heart attack. All certainty eroded. All carefree days ended. She hadn't signed up for this – heart attacks, uncertainty and fear. We had so much left to do. That's what the vegan diet, abstaining from alcohol and exercising every day were for. They were to make sure we still had time to do everything we wanted to do. But something had changed in me after the heart attack. I'd become more impatient, less forgiving, a little bitter even. I would watch people happily quaffing their beer and wine at the pub and I would resent them. I would stare at fellow diners in our local restaurant as they tucked into their steak and chips and think, 'Why me?' But I already knew *why me*. The doctors had told me. I cursed my genes and stared at the screen again. How do you type a positive ending to your story when you are not sure the ending is positive? But I wasn't sure the ending was negative either. I hadn't been diagnosed with anything yet. So, until I knew for certain I had cancer I would be better off ignoring the possibility entirely.

So that's exactly what I did. I threw myself into my work and completing the memoir, with all the passion and drive I could muster, while all the while this nagging fear that I might have cancer just murmured incessantly in the back of my head. The real beauty of the writing was that I could totally immerse myself in it. Get lost in the story. Laugh and cry at the moments of my life that had scarred me, shaped me and made me. And suspend the reality of the present moment and what might be coming down the line.

What was coming was an MRI. A noisy and nerve-wracking affair. The results came back quickly but didn't really help much. They didn't indicate cancer, nor did they suggest whatever had shown up in my prostate was benign either. Instead, they came back as 'inconclusive'. Not very helpful at all really. Another blood test showed my PSA had risen again and was now at a very inconvenient 10.4. Both results were enough for the thorough, and still annoyingly concerned, Dr Alderton, to firmly recommend a template biopsy. He explained what it entailed, and I wished he hadn't bothered. A general anaesthetic followed by an ultrasound up my back passage and several needles into my perineum – the area between my testicles and bum. My eyes watered at the thought of it. Carefree fun-filled days definitely long gone. Replaced now by fingers and devices up my bottom at all too regular intervals.

It was biopsy day. It all felt too soon. Geraldine sat with me in the waiting room, on Ward 4, of the Freeman Hospital. Yes, it all felt too soon since it was less than three years since I'd been rushed here with a 99 per cent blockage in my left anterior descending artery, the 'widow-maker' artery, so-called because a blockage there is one of the deadliest heart attacks to have. Without emergency treatment survival is virtually impossible. But I had gotten emergency treatment. I'd gotten it here in this very hospital. I'd changed my lifestyle completely because of it. I'd done that because I never again wanted to be a patient here but, less than three years later, here I was, regardless. A patient once more, staring vacantly at the TV screen in the corner of the day room, trying to lip read the newsreader as the volume was off. Geraldine held my hand and sat in silence. She'd given up on the small talk when she'd stopped getting any response 20 minutes earlier. I didn't look at her as I spoke.

'I'm really sorry I'm putting you through this again. I don't want this to be happening so soon after the heart stuff.'

She squeezed my hand.

'Don't be so stupid. It can't be helped.'

I gripped her hand tightly. I thought about the last three years, about how our lives had changed. All of our plans for growing old together felt like they crumbled away overnight. In the weeks and months of fear and uncertainty that followed, it was like I was a different person entirely to who I'd been before. Because of that we were different. We no longer made long term plans. Yes, we planned next year's holiday, or for when our children would leave home and we would be left in our empty nest. But the heart attack hung over our lives like a dark cloud. My change of lifestyle was my attempt to fight back, to take back some sort of control, and bring the sunshine back. I just wanted us to get to where we were before, to the life I'd taken for granted. But I knew it was changed forever, and most likely would be shorter than I'd ever imagined it would be. I wanted to get it all back for her more than me. She was someone who had never complained, or showed a flicker of disappointment or fear, but instead, just got on with whatever it was that life had thrown at us over the years, including the heart attack. But now, here, waiting for her husband to undergo a biopsy to determine whether or not we could add cancer to our life's journey, I suddenly felt very sorry for her. She should have been in class today teaching her group of noisy three- and four-year-olds. Watching them run, skip and jump their way through an energetic lunch break. I thought of my own childhood, scarred by The Troubles in Northern Ireland. My innocence robbed early by my mother Bernadette's heart attack when I was just five years old. I'd become aware of death, or the fear of death, far too early in my short existence. But in the last three years it had gone from being an irritant at the back of my mind to something that dominated my every thought. I had to fight it every day, the fear that I could have died from my heart attack without the intervention I'd received in the same hospital I now sat in again. That's hard to live with. The most difficult thing to cope with was the knowledge that outside of your immediate family, the rest of the world just didn't seem to care. So, after my heart attack and even now, with the tests for cancer, I just hadn't talked to anyone about it. Anyone, except the warm kind girl that I'd fallen in love with so long ago, who now held my hand too tightly as we sat in the tired sterile waiting room, staring at an old TV with the volume switched off.

I wanted better for her. I wanted holidays, happiness, love and laughter. Instead, what I'd given her was insecurity, fear, uncertainty and heartache. What I'd hidden from the world she witnessed in all its aching fragility – the disappearance of my health, the shattering of my confidence in the future, and the birth of a new *me*. I was acutely aware I was utterly changed from the man I'd been only three years before. It was small things to begin with; turning down an invitation here and there; not being able to get myself off the chair in the evenings; some days not wanting to go to work. It went all the way to *what's the fucking point?* I didn't want to be that person. I'd fought hard against my descent. But days like today were tough ones to take. As the round nurse with the red face approached me to take me to the pre-op ward, I was definitely at *what's the fucking point* again. I kissed Geraldine. I told her everything would be fine. *Everything is always going to be fine.*

'No point in you hanging around here. Go on home and I will call you when I'm done.'

But she didn't leave. She came with me as I morphed from me into the patient in Bay 2. Ready to be poked, prodded and questioned until it was my time. After several hours, she was fighting to keep her eyes open and shuffling uncomfortably on her wooden chair while I lay in bed waiting to be called for my biopsy. We'd been in the hospital since 7.30 a.m. and it was approaching 2 p.m. She sat up, yawned and squinted at her watch.

'Christ… it's 2 o'clock. Why did we need to be here at half-seven if they weren't going to take you till now? I will have to go and get Ciaran from school.'

I felt a pang of guilt. *Ciaran*.

Ciaran was the youngest of our three boys. He was 12 when I'd suffered my heart attack. I'd lied to him about it. Not told him. I didn't want him to worry. I didn't want to shatter his innocence. When I eventually told him the truth, he'd made me promise there would be no more lies, no more secrets. Yet here I was again back in hospital and he didn't know. In fact, none of them knew. Owen and Conor, too, were getting on with their day, blissfully unaware that their father's health, or lack of it, was back on the agenda. I was meeting Owen the following day to pick up the birthday cake we'd ordered for the surprise 50th birthday party I'd organised for Geraldine the day after that. *The party!*

I'd barely given it a thought over the past 24 hours but planning it and making sure all of her family and mine were flying in from Ireland had been a welcome distraction and had kept my mind off biopsies and cancer for the last few weeks. I was a little worried that it was happening just two days after my perineum was to be punctured multiple times, but there was nothing much I could do about the timing.

Geraldine left to get Ciaran. A very kind nurse, with a wealth of experience in talking to men about their nether regions, explained the procedure and its aftermath. Blood in the urine and semen were the main bits I remembered. That, and that I would have a sore bottom for a few days, like there was a golf ball lodged in there. I would have my results in a week or two. A birthday party, in two days' time, suddenly felt like I might be pushing it a bit.

I awoke from the anaesthetic. The more it wore off, the more it became very apparent that my surgeon had replaced the golf ball with something else altogether. It felt like he had shoved a tennis ball up my bum. The party would certainly be interesting.

CHAPTER 7

Thankfully, my tennis ball had shrunk to a golf ball by the time Geraldine's birthday came around on 8 December 2016. That encouraged us to try and celebrate it in the old-fashioned way – by making love. We had an hour before I was due to pick up various members of the family from the airport. Geraldine had some time before she would be summoned to pick up Owen from university, all part of the plan to get her out of the house, so that I could sneak the family in. I was enjoying myself so much I'd forgotten all about the nurse's words after my biopsy. That was until I felt the first spasms in my golf ball. I looked down just in time to see thick black blood erupt from me. It was like watching a pornographic horror film. Is that even a genre? *God, I hope not!*

My golf ball was still spasming and twitching as I sat in the airport car park. Thankfully the painkillers had made the drive bearable. Visions of thick black semen oozing from my penis were still swirling around my head as I transported my family back to the house. I did my best to join in the excited chatter but spent the 20-minute journey with my stomach churning at the thought of this morning's events. Geraldine's reaction when she came home to discover her mum and dad, sister Caroline and her husband David, and my sister Denise and my brother-in-law Kieran, all siting in our living room, finally helped banish the horror porn from my head.

The joy and atmosphere of the day was in stark contrast to how it had begun. The whole family spent the day at the Christmas market in Newcastle and the evening at our favourite bistro in Wylam. Apart from the constant throbbing in my bottom, it was as if nothing was the matter, and all was good in our world. We extended the night with a party back at our house, and that too, was going well, until a tipsy Geraldine began to speak. Her intention was to thank everybody for coming and making her 50th birthday so special. She looked at me and started to thank me for organising the event. I could see her eyes fill with tears before she got her first words out. She stuttered, she stammered, and then she began to cry uncontrollably. I leaned over and she threw her arms around my neck.

'I love you so much. I don't want to…'

I let go of her and stared into her eyes red from crying, and shook my head. She composed herself. I looked around the room. It must have seemed such an exaggerated reaction from her to what, after all, was no big effort from me. I had only organised a few flights and a meal in a restaurant. I was glad that she steadied herself before speaking again.

'I just want to say how much I love my husband and I want to thank him for the life we have tog…'

Her arms were back around my neck and she was soaking my shirt and heaving uncontrollably into my chest. I held her as she let out everything she had kept in. When she had calmed herself and let go, I studied the confused faces of our family, raised my eyebrows, and passed Geraldine a napkin.

'No more Prosecco for you!'

She laughed and apologised.

'Sorry, I'm just getting sentimental in my old age. But everyone I care about most in the world is in this room and I want you all to know how much I appreciate you coming. I want to thank Paul for…'

I could hear her voice breaking and decided to intervene to prevent a third crying fit. I started a chorus of 'happy birthday' and by the time we'd finished, Geraldine had aborted all attempts at thanking me for organising her birthday celebrations. Her emotion hadn't gone unnoticed though.

'Is everything alright with Geraldine?'

Her father, Leo, was nursing his drink and leaning against the kitchen sink. He was a quiet man. Never one to make a fuss, but like all fathers he didn't like to see his daughter so upset. As father-in-law's go, he was a very good one. I can't remember ever having a cross word with him since I first sat on his settee as a nervous spotty 15-year-old. He was in his late 70s now and his health, both mental and physical, was all too obviously in steep decline. A heart attack and a quadruple bypass at 49 had taken their toll and early dementia had opened a door to constant confusion, irritability and endless repeated conversations.

I filled his glass and leaned on the sink next to him.

'She's great. I just think she is a bit overwhelmed that you all made it across – especially you. I don't think she expected to see you here again with your health troubles.'

He was never a man to show too much emotion. So what came next took me by complete surprise. I could hear the tremor in his voice as he spoke quietly to me.

'She's a special one Geraldine. One of a kind. I couldn't be prouder of her.'

He stared intently across the room to where his eldest daughter was deep in conversation with my sister Denise. I spoke without looking at him.

'She is that, Leo. She's made me very happy in my life, and she is a great mother to the kids as well. We have been very happy.'

I felt his frail hand on top of mine.

'I wanted to say, son, how proud I am of you, and I want to thank you for looking after my daughter. I couldn't have asked for a better son-in-law than you. I know you will always look after her.'

His voice had broken half-way through the sentence and by the time he had finished, he was dabbing his eyes with the handkerchief that old people always seem to have, no matter what the occasion.

'What are you two talking about?'

Geraldine had made her way across the kitchen and was linking us all together.

I squeezed her arm.

'What do you think?'

The three of us stood in silence. Nothing to say but just *be*. I wondered what was going on inside her head as she held onto her frail father and fragile husband. Her efforts at speaking earlier had given me a fair idea. I kept a watchful eye on her for the rest of the night in case of any further attempts at prematurely revealing what we had been dealing with over the past few weeks.

* * *

Ollie ran ahead as we struggled up the hill. It was a few days after the party. The air was cold and crisp, and our breath was a cloud around us. My golf ball was now a marble and not troubling me at all, unless I sat on it. But if my marble wasn't troubling me, then *So You Did* certainly was. Not the memoir itself, just the title. I had almost finished it, and while I was happy with the contents, the title just didn't seem to fit it somehow. Geraldine had come up with several alternatives and I had done the same. We were nearing the top of the tree-lined hill and Ollie was darting in and out of sight and going wherever his nose took him. Geraldine stopped. I strode on.

'Come on lazy. I need this for my heart.'

She didn't move. I walked back to her.

'I've got it.'

'Got what?'

'The title of the book.'

She'd given me so many titles most of which I'd thought were complete rubbish, that I wasn't hopeful that her eureka moment was going to yield anything of any note. As soon as she spoke, I knew she had found the perfect title.

'*The Boy on the Shed*. You should call it *The Boy on the Shed*. It's perfect. You used to spend all your time up there watching over your mum when she was ill. It is a…'

I put my finger over her lips.

'Stop. Stop selling it to me.'

She pushed my hand away.

'But it's perfect. *The Boy on the Shed. The Boy on the Shed. The Boy on the Shed.* Don't you get it? It's better than anything you've come up with and more appropriate than *So You Did.*'

I feigned a lack of enthusiasm for her brilliant suggestion. She was getting annoyed. That was something that happened so seldom, that I let her get a little more irate before intervening.

'OK, OK! I agree! It's perfect. *The Boy on the Shed.* I love it. That's the title. Thank you. It's fantastic. Now I just need to finish it and we need to find an agent and a publisher to print the thing.'

I did finish it. I finished it that afternoon sitting at my dining room table looking out over the garden. Geraldine busied herself in the kitchen while waiting to read the final chapter. I could barely feel the marble now and I knew nothing of what was to come with the impending diagnosis. I might have cancer, but then again, I might not. So I wrote what I felt were the perfect five words to encapsulate how I was feeling. *It is only autumn still.* There was a lot more life left in me yet. I also had my cardiology appointment coming up later in the week and I knew I was doing all I could to make sure I didn't suffer another *event.* I had no idea when I would get the results of the biopsy, but most likely it would be a few weeks off.

I handed Geraldine the laptop and swapped places with her in the kitchen. She made her way into the living room to read my final words. She'd been my editor all the way through the process. I would write a chapter sitting opposite her at the kitchen or dining room table and then pass it to her for comment and corrections. All the way through she had been incredibly positive about the story and how I'd written it. In places, if I was wracked with doubt, she would quickly dismiss my concerns and tell me how good she thought the writing was. She'd laughed in the right places, and cried in the right places, too. Now as the kettle boiled behind me, I tried to peer around the living room door to catch a glimpse of her reading the final chapter on the settee.

'What are you doing dad?'

Ciaran was standing behind me, looking over my shoulder and into the living room.

I shushed him.

'I'm trying to watch your mum reading the final chapter of my book. But I don't want her to see me.'

I stepped out of the way.

'You have a look for me. She'll be less suspicious of you peeping at her.'

He shook his head but did his duty. I poured the hot water into the cups. He was back behind me.

'Dad. She's crying. Do you want me to go and see what's wrong?'

I smiled at him.

'Is she sniffling, sobbing or crying?'

He went back to check. He came back concerned and confused.

'She's crying, like really crying Dad.'

I patted him on the shoulder.

'That's great son. Really great.'

He shook his head again.

'You're weird as fu…you're really weird dad.'

And with that, he headed off to the sanctuary of his bedroom. I carried Geraldine's tea into the living room. She was still crying as she spoke.

'It's really, really good Paul. In fact, it's brilliant. I loved the last line. I loved the whole thing. You should be really proud of it. Even if you never get a publisher. The kids and their kids will have a record of who we are and where they come from, and that will be a precious thing for them someday. We sat in silence and stared at *The Boy on the Shed*. It would probably never be read by anyone outside of our family, but I was proud of it and glad I'd written it. I was particularly pleased with the closing line.

* * *

We sat in the car for what seemed like an eternity. We hadn't spoken since we'd left Dr Alderton's office. I thought about the birthday party we'd had only days ago, then of sitting beside Geraldine, drinking tea and celebrating the completion of *The Boy on the Shed*. I thought about the struggle of the last three years to bring some normality back to our life after the heart attack. I thought about the uncertainty of the last few weeks – MRI scans, biopsies and bloody semen. Dr Alderton's soul-crushing words echoed around my head. Then, finally, I thought about the boys. My three children, who were no longer children. I thought about having to speak with them, to tell them their dad had cancer. I thought about the fear and uncertainty that would bring to their young lives. Then I started to cry.

CHAPTER 8

I'd heard people talk about the moment they were diagnosed with cancer. I'd heard them describe it as a life-changing event, a hammer blow, how life as they'd known it altered forever. There was life before cancer and life after cancer. There is no doubt that by the time I'd composed myself enough to get out of the car park and begin the journey home I felt like everything in my life had changed. All the tests and the positive conversations with Geraldine of what we would do if the diagnosis was cancer just faded into nothingness. All the talk of 'dealing with whatever comes' meant nothing to me. I felt like my world had closed in around my ears the moment Dr Alderton delivered the bad news, inadvertently blocking my path to Geraldine as he did so. I was listening to him after that but none of it really landed with me. I registered 'bone scans', 'cancer in both lobes', 'surgery best option', 'hormone therapy and radiotherapy', 'incontinence', 'erectile dysfunction' and 'life limiting'. I'm sure he was speaking in perfectly constructed sentences and was making complete sense to everyone else in the room, but to me he was obliterating my future right there in his brightly lit office. Who wants to be told they have prostate cancer? Who wants the Hobson's choice of a surgical removal of the prostate gland (prostatectomy), or hormone treatment and radiotherapy, with incontinence and erectile dysfunction the likely side effects of both? Certainly not me. Not at 51 years old. It was bad enough spewing dark grainy blood out of my erect penis on Geraldine's birthday, but that was infinitely better than producing absolutely nothing out of a permanently flaccid one. Who would have thought a bit of cancer in one little gland could potentially be so life altering? Then there was the bone scan I needed in order to establish if the cancer had already spread beyond my prostate. In which case, the surgical option and any hope of a cure was off the agenda. A stupid little gland that was now in danger of blowing my entire life right off course. A little walnut, that most men including me, didn't fully understand or appreciate. I had friends who called it 'prostrate' cancer. If only. If I had 'prostrate' cancer, then I could just stand up and that would make it all miraculously disappear. I'd never lie down again.

But I didn't have 'prostrate' cancer, I had prostate cancer and by the time I pulled up outside our house it was giving me a headache. Literally. Right between my eyes. I had a pounding headache and felt sick as I entered the house. Geraldine put the kettle on. I threw up in the bathroom. My mind raced between the thought of having cancer and the thought of telling my three boys I had cancer. The thought of speaking with them made my knees weak, my palms moist and my mouth dry. I was sick of dropping bombs into their young lives.

'You have to tell them sooner rather than later. You are going to be having surgery or other treatment, you won't be well. You can't keep things like this to yourself. It's not a cut on your knee or an upset stomach.'

We were sitting in semi-darkness in our living room. Geraldine was making complete sense as usual. But the dread of telling the boys was overwhelming me.

'I'm not even sure I could speak to them without getting upset. I don't want to upset them. Do you want to tell them?'

She was shaking her head before I'd finished.

'That would be worse for them. You tell them and reassure them that everything will be alright. They'll cope. They're strong and dealt with your heart attack. They'll deal with this too.'

She was right in her logic but it proved to be a mistake in the end. That afternoon, after I'd composed myself enough, I attempted to speak to each of them individually and in person. I was calm and collected on every occasion, until I got to the point where I had to tell them that I had prostate cancer. No matter how hard I tried, I simply couldn't get the words out without a rush of emotion from my gut spilling out through my eyes. I no doubt made the situation much more worrying for all of them. Who wants to see their father blubbing and crying in front of you at any time, never mind when he is telling you he has cancer and trying to convince you everything is going to be alright in the end?

That night we all met up for dinner. It wasn't planned. Well, not by me anyway. Me, Geraldine and Ciaran visited a little Italian restaurant where we had often gone as a family when the boys were younger and still living at home. Owen was at university now and living in the city, while Conor had his own place with Kayleigh, who was seven months pregnant with our first grandchild. We no longer just popped out as a family for a mid-week meal. Those days were gone, and I missed them so much. But tonight, not long after the three of us sat down, we got a call from Conor. He just happened to be around the corner and could join us. Five minutes later Owen, by coincidence, was shopping nearby.

As the main courses arrived, I looked around the table at the boys who were now young men. It was such a familiar scene to me. I'd shared this table with them since they had all been in high-chairs. I'd ordered for them, cut their food up for them, looked after their every need. But tonight was different. They didn't need me anymore. But I needed them. I needed them more than I had needed them in my entire life… and they were here. I could feel my stomach tighten and my chest following it. I excused myself as the waiter arrived with the food. I'd barely made it to the bathroom cubicle when the tears came again in a flood. The boys had seen enough of their father blubbing for one day. My pasta was cold by the time I'd got back to the table. We talked about Ciaran's school, Owen's university and the impending birth of Conor's daughter. We talked about Christmas and the summer holiday to Italy we were planning. We talked about old times and new times to come. We didn't talk about my failing health, heart disease, or cancer. When dinner was over, we hugged as always. I held each of them a little tighter for a little longer.

After the initial shock, life trundled along as normal. There were lots of restless nights, too much Googling, and turning down invitations to go out with friends. But life doesn't stop after a cancer diagnosis. You might well be in turmoil on the inside, but the world outside doesn't miss a beat. That fact in itself can make you feel incredibly lonely. You can be in the middle of a busy office, sitting on a train, or laughing on a night out with friends, but inside you are lost, alone and terrified of the uncertain future to come. But bills needed to be paid and work had to be done. As the CEO of Speedflex, I couldn't just lock myself away from the world and lick my wounds at home. Which was a good thing in many ways, because that's exactly what I wanted to do. Go and hide from everything and everybody I knew. Withdraw from it all and never come back. If I'd been allowed to do what I wanted to do, I would've very rapidly disappeared into a black hole that I would never have been able to get out of again. I'm glad that it just wasn't an option for me. Instead, I turned up for work every day, tried my best to think about the task in front of me, rather than the upcoming flurry of appointments and activity that would lead me inevitably to surgery or hormone treatment and radiotherapy, and all the life-altering side effects that every route guaranteed. But it's hard to pretend all is well when it isn't, at least for me. I struggled to keep up appearances of normality. My mask would occasionally slip, usually manifesting itself in an exaggerated response to a small problem at work, or a snap at a colleague who'd just asked a perfectly reasonable question. That irritability was evident at home too. I would pick an argument with Geraldine or Ciaran where it was entirely unnecessary, and then hate myself as I'd watch them look back at me confused and helpless and unable to defend themselves for fear of making the situation worse. My mental turmoil manifested itself in self-sabotage of my recent exemplary fitness regime. Junk food, still vegan, but junk food nevertheless, became my comfort. I exercised less and ate more. My weight began to creep back on and before I knew it, I was a stone heavier than the day only weeks before when I'd sat with Dr Alderton and he'd confirmed my diagnosis. There would be moments when I would forget all about it, but they were short respites. It felt like every time I opened the mailbox, it would contain an appointment letter or a correspondence between doctors outlining the treatment options based on my last visit to the hospital. The condition always looked worse on paper. During a consultation, there was always the comfort of the surgeon talking positively about the prognosis and the treatments available to me. Seeing the words on a page, bold and black, discussing Mr Ferris's cancer was always a punch in the stomach, a dose of stark reality.

The appointments themselves seemed to be coming thick and fast, too, just to make sure I couldn't settle back into normal life. My next one was with the oncologist. I don't think I'd even met an -*ologist* until my heart attack and now I was spending far too much time with them. If you are sharing your day with -*ologists,* then take it from me that is not a good day. Unless of course you are learning to be a bird watcher, or maybe about to have a baby or… never mind… you get the picture. I wasn't studying birds and certainly not having a baby, but -*ologists* were everywhere.

My latest one was sitting in front of me. Dr Frew was a very pleasant Scotsman from the borders. We discussed my biopsy results and my prognosis – and whether I should choose the surgical route, or radiotherapy and hormone treatment. He was very thorough in his outlining of the side effects of both. They were basically the same no matter what route I chose. I wasn't getting out of this one without regularly wetting myself, and my chances of getting erections without the support of medication or scaffolding were remote too. You would think that after nearly 30 years of marriage that the thought of having no erections wouldn't bother me so much, but it did. It really did. Every time Dr Frew mentioned it, or Dr Alderton before him, I felt my stomach flip and my mouth dry up. If I had the surgery, then Dr Alderton would perform laparoscopic surgery through a series of incisions in my abdomen. He'd guide robotic arms as they removed my prostate from my body, without damaging the delicate nerves to my penis, and giving me a better chance of having erections again. If I chose the radiotherapy route, Dr Frew would not put me on the usual two-year hormone treatment plan as this would kill any interest I had in sex, whether I had an erection or not. Because I was still relatively young, I would have six months of hormone treatment instead. This was to ensure I was left with some sort of libido on the other side of my treatment. With the surgery, I would have the satisfaction of knowing that the cancer had been cut out and my PSA would immediately go down to a negligible level. With the radiotherapy, I wouldn't get that instant drop but rather a gradual decrease in PSA. I might get some permanent bowel damage from the radiation, but that might not present itself until sometime after the treatment. I would have to self-administer daily enemas during the radiotherapy process and there was a very small risk of other cancers developing as a result of my treatment. There was a third option – a six-week clinical trial, that involved greater doses of radiation administered over a much shorter timeframe, but its effectiveness and potential side effects were not fully understood. I really liked Dr Frew. In another life, and in different circumstances, he would have been a friend of mine. I was so impressed with him that by the time I'd left his office, I was asking the receptionist for the clinical trial form, so that I could sign up for his six-week experiment.

But an hour of talking the whole thing through with Geraldine that evening convinced me that what I really wanted was my cancerous prostate cut out. I wanted it cut out as quickly as possible, so that I could be cured and get on with my life. Admittedly, it was a life where I may end up wetting myself into pads and very probably saying goodbye to erections. The potential side effects of surgery (which were the same for radiotherapy and hormone treatment) seemed irrelevant at that moment. Getting rid of the cancer was all that mattered to me.

CHAPTER 9

Christmas 2016, and the imminent arrival of our first grandchild, brought a much-needed semblance of normality to my life. I threw myself into the preparations as I always did – it's my favourite time of the year. I love all of it – the lights, the music, the food and drink, but most of all, the sentiment. I love the romance of Christmas, the family feel of it and the nostalgia, too. It often transports me back to my childhood days in Ireland. I can still vividly remember bouncing down the stairs one Christmas morning aged five, being greeted by my father stoking the fire in the living room while singing Neil Diamond's *Cracklin' Rosie* at the top of his voice. All felt good in my world that day. I was happy, I was safe, and I was loved. *Soley Soley* by Middle of the Road was playing on the radio, my mother was busy preparing a breakfast of bacon, eggs and soda bread, and Santa had been. It was a magical Christmas morning I will never forget. My mother had suffered her first heart attack that year. It had rocked my foundations. But she was home from hospital now. We had breakfast squashed on the tiny settee in front of the roaring fire. Just the three of us. No one else was up. I had them all to myself. We hadn't needed to be so squashed. We did have other chairs in the room. But I hadn't waited for a second invitation from my mother to squeeze my bony frame in between them both. It was the best place in the world to be. A perfect start to any Christmas Day.

That wasn't the case every year. Once, I came downstairs and found Brendan O'Neill, my boyhood friend, already in our sitting room, playing happily with a new crane Santa had brought me. *Playing with my toys before I'd had a chance to!* He ended up getting momentarily strangled, before my mother clipped me around the ear and made me apologise. There was often a war on Christmas Day. The worst by far was when I accidently put my foot through my brother Tony's drum kit. He retaliated by eating my Subbuteo balls. *Both of them!* Toy thieves and ball-eaters aside, I've always loved Christmas. I even used to like going to mass at Christmas. But only if it was midnight mass on Christmas Eve. The excitement of the day to follow made up for the boring hour spent in the company of perfectly dressed families and foul-smelling drunks, who had made their way from all-day drinking sessions at the pub. Our midnight mass, at St Patrick's Church in Lisburn, was brought forward to 9 p.m. on Christmas Eve, to encourage the former and discourage the latter. It didn't work. The first year it was changed, I made my way into the pew and knelt right in the middle of a pile of steaming vomit courtesy of the sleeping drunk slumped next to me. On some years, Santa's presents were a little suspect – blue space hoppers and pogo sticks that didn't spring. None of those minor irritations could dampen my enthusiasm for Christmas. The first whispers of John and Yoko's *Happy Xmas (War is Over)*, would get me right in the middle of my chest. It still does, every time I hear it, more than 50 years after they recorded it. The Pogue's *Fairytale of New York* does the same to me. The first bars on the piano and I'm off in Christmas bliss every single time. Well maybe not exactly every single time. Not this year.

This year was different. *Fairytale of New York* doesn't sound so good when it is being played on the radio behind the deserted counter of The Nuclear Medicine Department at the Freeman Hospital.

'Enjoy your Christmas and we can pick this up with a bone scan in the New Year.'

They were the words of Dr Alderton when I'd told him I'd decided to have my prostate removed and he could cut the cancer out of me once and for all. But somebody at the Bone Scanning Centre was clearly more efficient than he'd expected, and I found myself trudging through the Northern Centre for Cancer Care and standing with Geraldine at the empty reception desk on the 23 December. This Christmas was certainly not going into the memory bank alongside *Cracklin' Rosie*, choking Brendan O'Neill, and losing my balls.

Geraldine rang the bell again as Shane McGowan's bells were ringing out for Christmas Day. A very sick, pencil-thin woman sat dozing next to an equally sick 40-year-old Christmas tree. She may well have been younger than the tree, but whatever horrible condition she was suffering from made the poor woman look much older. No one came, so we sat in silence as Shane gave way to Wizzard's *I Wish it Could be Christmas Every Day*, which sounded horribly out of place.

'Sorry to have kept you waiting. Mr Ferris, is it?'

A smiling face was now standing behind the reception. She was round and ruddy. As I approached, I could smell the alcohol she'd just consumed, before returning to her post.

'It's all gone a bit Christmassy here I'm afraid. Our colleague is leaving as well, so we are having a bit of a do for her. You are the last patient before Christmas. The radiographer will be with you shortly.'

She sat down, expertly unwrapped a purple Quality Street and sang along to Wizzard, as I made my way back to Geraldine. I was all out of Christmas spirit.

'Why the fuck have they booked me a bone scan for 23rd of December? They won't be able to give me the results until after Christmas anyway. Couldn't they have just waited until after Christmas, so I can enjoy *Cracklin' Rosie* and choking Brendan? Now I'm going to have a scan to establish whether or not the cancer has spread to my bones but will have no idea of the results for weeks, months maybe.'

She took my hand.

'Calm down. They are only trying to help. Now, let's get it done and we can get on with *Cracklin' Rosie* and choking Brendan. We have a granddaughter due in days and our family will all be here for

Christmas. This is just something to get out of the way. Then we can go and enjoy ourselves.'

I was thinking that I needed to update my Christmas stories when the radiographer called me through. She injected me with dye, and five minutes later I was back in time for the radio to ruin my decades of warm feelings towards John and Yoko. They were whispering from behind the reception desk. I wasn't feeling it from them this year. We left the sick tree and sick woman and headed into town to pass the three hours required for the dye to work its way through my bones, so that the radiographer had the best chance of identifying any tumours that had possibly migrated there. Were she to find any, then my prognosis would suddenly become much more bleak. That was the thought that occupied me as we made our way through the Christmas market in the city centre. Not the carol singers, or the smell of bratwurst and macaroons, but what the future held if the cancer had already spread beyond my prostate. Not the most festive thought I've ever had on the 23 December.

I was still thinking that thought, while lying under the scanner three hours later, and still thinking it, when the cheery radiographer came back into the room to tell me it was all done. I knew the answer to my question before asking it but asked it all the same. I had to. It was the only thing on my mind and the only thing that mattered in my life at that moment.

'Did you see anything on the scan?'

I was annoyed with myself for asking. I only did so because I had scared myself half to death, telling myself that the tone of her voice was different to when she had injected the dye three hours previously, and when she had put me on the slab 30 minutes ago. *She knew something. She'd seen something. She was hiding something.* If she did know something, had seen something, and was hiding something, she did a pretty good job of concealing it, as she guided me off the hard surface.

'Sorry Mr Ferris, I just work the scanner. I haven't even looked at it and I'm not the person who analyses it. You will find out after Christmas and I hope you get the results you are looking for.'

That was it right there. The sentence that ruined Christmas 2016. *I hope you get the results you are looking for.* John Lennon and Shane McGowan could fuck off this Christmas. I wasn't in the mood for them, and they could take Roy Wood with them.

The great big world we live in exists entirely between our ears. I learned that truth many years ago. The stories we tell ourselves, how we think, how we interact with others, all of it, is there within us for us to shape and mould in any way we see fit. We are in control of our minds and not the other way around. When we live in the moment and choose to be happy then we are happy. *What a complete load of bollox!*

When it's Christmas Eve, and you have just found out you have prostate cancer, and you are thumbing through the booklet on life-changing side effects that will be with you even if the treatment is successful, life feels pretty shit. When it's Christmas Day and you are looking around at the smiling faces of the people you care about most in the world but all the while fretting about the results of a bone scan that will determine how many more times you can share this experience with them, life feels pretty shit. All the self-help, self-improvement, inspirational books and quotes you read when you are in a good place seem so profound at the time and I can remember reading some of them and thinking I had discovered the answers to all my problems. I lost my Catholic faith many years ago. Indeed, I lost my faith in any higher power. There was just too much evidence to the contrary to continue to follow the myth. But I had read a lot of new-age spiritualist writing too. I suppose none of us really stop searching to try and make sense of the cosmic accident we appear to be. *Put good thoughts out into the universe and the universe will deliver your every wish. More bollox!*

It's hard to live in the moment, tell yourself you're happy, put positive thoughts out anywhere, never mind into the universe, when all certainty in your life is crumbling away. As I sat eating my fake turkey, while my family devoured the real turkey, the presence of one person at the table, or should I say two people, was the only thing that kept me from leaving the table, going upstairs, climbing into bed and cancelling Christmas. Her name was Kayleigh, and up until very recently she had been a stranger to me. But today she sat at the head of our table, next to my son Conor. She was naturally shy, and I could see she was a little uncomfortable. It wasn't just because she was sharing her Christmas lunch with me, Geraldine and our boys, instead of with her own family. No, she was uncomfortable too because of her growing belly. It was forcing her to sit so far back from the table that she could hardly reach her food. Inside it, was precious cargo, and the only positive thing that was happening in my life this Christmas. She and Conor had not been going out long when she had fallen pregnant. She'd sat nervously in our living room when they'd told us the news. I'd made her a promise that from that day forwards, whatever happened between her and Conor, we would always be there for her and her baby to come. I had meant every word. Once we had gotten over the shock, the thought of having our first grandchild was a great thrill for Geraldine and me. It was a long time since we'd sat on a bus to Belfast, making teenage plans about our future family together. It was also nearly 30 years since my beloved mother Bernadette had left me. When we found out halfway through the pregnancy that we were to have a granddaughter, it really did feel like the universe was granting my wishes. *Never mind the bollox!*

The imminent arrival of our granddaughter was the only thought that banished the fear that consumed me over the Christmas of 2016. I couldn't wait for her arrival. Thankfully I didn't have to wait long. Kayleigh went into labour on Boxing Day and gave birth on the following morning. As I walked towards the ward to meet her for the first time, I had to take several deep breaths and steady myself on my trembling legs. I knew something very special had just happened and someone very precious had just come into my life. I picked up the tiny bundle and brought it to my face. I kissed her gently on the head and whispered in her unhearing ear.

'Hello beautiful. I'm your Granda, and you've no idea how glad I am that you chose to arrive at this time. You are a very special girl.'

Isla's presence in my world hit me in my chest and cleared the fog between my ears. She instantly dampened the fear and gave me hope for the future. Maybe the universe really had intervened after all.

CHAPTER 10

As I toasted the New Year of 2017, I was in a much better place than I'd been for the Christmas celebrations. The arrival of Isla on the 27th had been quickly followed by some great news on the 28th. Julie Needham, the Speedflex member who'd now become my nurse, rang to let me know that the bone scans had come back negative. I had prostate cancer, but it was localised to my prostate, and that meant everything in terms of my prognosis. I had early-stage cancer that could be cured. I was grateful for her kindness in making the call during the Christmas holidays. If she hadn't, I probably wouldn't have heard the good news until well into the New Year.

I began to realise that while it wasn't ideal to have cancer on top of heart disease that I was, in fact, luckier than a lot of others who had suffered from one or the other. The reality was that I'd suffered a heart attack, yet it hadn't killed me. Now, I was being told that my cancer had been caught early enough to have a fighting chance of a cure. They were both things to be celebrated and tackled head-on rather than to be feared. I was on medication for my heart and now I could have my prostate cut out of me and the cancer would go with it. The birth of this little girl, felt like a precious gift at the perfect time. Life was by no means good; how could it be? But I could at least see that it could and would be good again. More importantly, I could visualise a future for my family where I was still a part of it.

My surgery was booked for early February. Isla's arrival ensured I had no time to worry about what was to come. We saw her as much as we possibly could, without making obvious nuisances of ourselves. Each time we did she just came to mean more and more to me. I'd read an American bumper sticker years ago that had made me laugh, but I'd never fully understood the sentiment until now. It read: 'If I'd had known having grandchildren was this good, I would have had them first.' I understood it completely now. Her tiny features, her delicate fingers, her smell, all intoxicated me and banished the thought of cancer and treatment completely from my head. Well, not completely. There was the constant dribbling and inability to pee properly to remind me every time I visited the bathroom. There was the interrupted sleep, and drowsy trudges back and forwards to the bathroom, while Geraldine slept soundly next to me. Then there were the pre-op protocols to follow. Calls from the specialist nurse to make sure I was mentally prepared for the life-changing effects of having my prostate pulled out through my belly button by a sophisticated robot operated by Dr Alderton.

Geraldine was reading the latest correspondence from the hospital. It was late in the evening in the middle of January. She started to laugh. Not the reaction I expected when she'd picked up the booklet entitled *How to Look After your Catheter*. I smiled at her.

'I'm glad my upcoming surgery is brightening up your night.'

She waved the thin booklet.

'I'm sorry. It's not funny. In fact, it's pretty grim, but this bit tickled me.'

She squinted over her glasses and sang aloud.

'The day bag's connected to the night bag. The night bag's connected to the day bag. The night bag's disconnected from the day bag, the day bag stays connected to the...'

She started laughing and handed me the booklet before heading off into the kitchen. I could hear her singing, 'The leg bone's connected to the knee bone, the knee bone's connected to the thigh bone, the thigh bone's connected to the hip bone...'

By the time she came back and filled my glass, she was on to the chorus. I began to read the instructions. I'd had the information for weeks but had just shoved it in the growing pile of hospital correspondence that was multiplying down by the side of my chair. I didn't want to read it until I really had to. With surgery now due in two weeks, I really couldn't put it off any longer. The rhyme that had amused Geraldine made for grim reading. It instantly soured my wine. I would have a catheter inserted during surgery, which I would then wear for a week. That was to ensure the stitches had healed, from where my urethra would be reattached to my bladder, after the removal of my prostate. The catheter itself was a tube that would be inserted up my penis, along my urethra, and into my bladder. Once there, a balloon would be inflated. My body might try to repel the catheter, and this could cause severe spasms and cramps. The tip of my penis would also become red and sore from having the tube inserted there, holding it permanently open. There were medications to help with the spasms and the stinging willy. Then there was the bit that had Geraldine singing *Dem Bones*. The tube would be connected to a day bag that would be strapped to my ankle. There would be a tap on that bag, so that I could empty it regularly. At night, when I was asleep, the night bag would be connected to the day bag, then the day bag… well you know the rest already. The day bag would stay on for five days. It would have a connection about six inches from the end of my penis. I was never to touch that during the five days, in case it led to infection.

By the time I'd finished reading about my surgery and catheter, not even scrolling through my latest photos of Isla could lift my mood. I opened my laptop and browsed the completed manuscript for *The Boy on the Shed*. Since I'd completed it, there was a new chapter in my life opening up. It was a bleak one. Geraldine was studying her phone when I interrupted her.

'Can we send this off to some agents?'

She sat her phone down.

'Yes. When do you want to send it off?'

I checked the time on my phone.

'Now, maybe?'

She glanced at the clock that hung behind my head.

'It's nearly half eight. Shouldn't we do it tomorrow, so we're not rushing it?'

I was already on a website that gave me a list of literary agents and their areas of interest. I needed to do it now. Tonight. To change the mood of the moment. She got off the settee and came and sat next to me. An hour later, we'd sent three chapters and a synopsis off to five agents. I'd done the same six years earlier with *An Irish Heartbeat*, the novel I'd written. I'm still waiting for a reply from any of them. So I didn't hold out much hope that this effort would be any different. But I needed to do it regardless. To do something to take my mind off the surgery to come. To have something positive to look forward to. When we had finished, I poured some wine and flicked through the TV channels in search of our latest binge watch. My phone buzzed beside my leg. I'd had an email response from an agent! It had only been 20 minutes since I'd sent the three chapters. I felt my chest flutter. This was the first contact I'd ever had from a literary agent. I could hardly stop my hand from shaking as I opened the email. My eyes raced across the text:

Thank you for your enquiry. Please note I am currently not taking submissions from new authors. Very best of luck in your search for an agent.'

I was just about to put the phone down when another email buzzed in. It could have been written by the same person. Two responses within seconds of each other, to inform me that *The Boy on the Shed* was facing the same fate as *An Irish Heartbeat*. At least this time I was getting responses, albeit standard rejections. I had only just put the phone down when the latest one came through. I assumed it was probably the same thing again:

Dear Paul,

What a wonderful surprise to receive on a Monday evening. I've read your three chapters and synopsis and think this represents a very exciting prospect. Could you please send me through the entire manuscript? Could I ask that you don't send it to any other literary agents until I have had a chance to read it and decide if I would like to

represent you? I would hope to give you an answer, one way or another,
by Friday.

   Yours faithfully,

   Guy Rose, Literary Agent.

   Futerman Rose and Associates

I couldn't even read it to Geraldine. My chest was thumping so much I was sure she could hear it. She read it and let out a squeal. Before long, two middle-aged idiots were hopping around the living room spilling wine on each other. After all, he'd only sent a request to read the manuscript, he might well do that and reject it out of hand. But it felt like something to hang on to, something to hope for. If he had liked the synopsis and three chapters so much and had got in touch within an hour, then there was no reason why he wouldn't like the rest of the manuscript surely? I composed myself enough to send him a very polite email. I pointed out that the manuscript was very raw and contained lots of typos and that I may have sent it off a little prematurely. I asked if he would give me a few days so that I could knock it into shape. I'd then send it to him by the weekend. I'd only just sent my stalling email off to him and he was back again. He didn't care about the typos, he just wanted to see the completed work. After more jumping around the living room, I sent it to him.

Three hours later, I was lying in bed and, for the first time, allowed myself to consider the possibility that in the middle of the mess I was in that I might actually one day be a published author. I thought of my mother, she'd died a lifetime ago when I was jobless and, but for the kindness of a friend, homeless too. Never in her wildest dreams would she have thought me capable of being a published author. Never in my wildest dreams would I have thought that either. It still might never happen, but at least there was a literary agent somewhere in the world who thought my writing good enough to at least consider it.

By the following morning, my nagging self-doubt had kicked in. What had I been thinking sending a manuscript full of typos to a literary agent? Why hadn't I just said no, and waited until I was happy with it, before sending it to him? It must have been the wine. He'd most probably be laughing over his coffee this morning at the quality of the writing and the uncorrected spelling mistakes. In my eagerness to get it off to him I'd probably blown my one and only chance to impress him. I was still kicking myself two days later when his email dropped into my inbox. I quickly scanned it for the gentle knock back:

'Thanks, but on reflection, and after wading through 100 spelling mistakes, and 200 typos, I've decided to pass on your rambling nonsense.'

But I didn't get that. In fact, what I got was so far away from that that I had to compose myself to read it again... and again... and again.

He loved the story. He loved the writing. He had no doubt whatsoever that he could find me a publisher. Not just any publisher, but one of the big ones like Hodder and Stoughton, Penguin, or Bloomsbury maybe. He would love nothing more than to represent me. If I agreed, he would send me a contract and start sending the manuscript off immediately.

I spent the rest of the day at work visualising *The Boy on the Shed* in the window of Waterstones and WH Smith, and at the top of Amazon's bestsellers' lists. I sent Guy an email that night confirming my agreement for him to represent me. I did mention that since completing the manuscript I had been diagnosed with prostate cancer and was about to have the diseased organ removed. I asked him if he thought I should add a further chapter at the end. He came back very quickly and told me to leave it as it was. There were enough traumas, emotion and life-changing events in there without dropping the reader 'off a cliff'. I took his advice, and by the Friday evening, I was now a prospective author, with my very own Literary Agent. I'd almost forgotten I was also a prospective author with prostate cancer. That was until the letter arrived on the following Saturday morning. It confirmed the exact date of my surgery. I was nervous about the upcoming operation, but happy that I'd soon be a prospective author who used to have prostate cancer. The side effects of the procedure were pretty gruesome, but I'd deal with them when I had to. I just wanted to get on with it now. Get the surgery done and get the cancer gone. The manuscript, the agent, and the potential book deal, were all very welcome distractions from what was hurtling my way.

CHAPTER 11

I arrived at the Freeman Hospital at 7 a.m. on a cold February morning in 2017. Geraldine sat with me for an hour until we found out my prostate wasn't going to be removed until late afternoon. What is it with hospitals and making sure you turn up eight hours before surgery? After a lot of persuasion and checking the contents of my bag for the tenth time, Geraldine left me so I could prepare for what was to come. Dr Alderton came to see me, and we had a discussion about the surgical procedure and the side effects. I think that day was the first time that I really allowed myself to think about the potential life-changing side effects of the surgery. It was a sobering thought to know that by the time I awoke, my body, and how it had served me up until that day, was never going to be the same again. But I was here now. No turning back. And it didn't matter how uncomfortable I felt about what he was telling me.

He was very thorough. I would spend up to four hours in surgery. He and his robot would make five incisions, including a large one in my belly button, through which my offending prostate would depart my body. I would wake up with a catheter in-situ and could expect to be in hospital for two or three days. The catheter would be removed after a week. Then, hopefully, I could expect to feel a lot better from that point onwards. He would spare the nerves. This should mean that I would eventually be able to have erections again sometime down the line. No guarantees though. I would also be incontinent. I would need to wear pads for a while until I recovered my ability to hold my own urine in. Finally, I could expect some shrinkage of my penis.

What? Jesus fucking Christ! Really?

He must have mentioned it before, but it was only there on the morning of my surgery, that this final indignity really hit home. When I awoke later that afternoon, I would no longer be able to have erections, or hold my urine in. Any orgasms in the future were likely to be far less pleasurable. I would never again produce semen. Now he was telling me my precious bits would be shrunk in size too!

Who the fuck in his right mind volunteers for surgery like this?

If it wasn't for what he wrote under the section headed 'Purpose of Operation' I may well have made my excuses and ducked out there and then. He wrote in large letters: TO CURE PROSTATE CANCER. As I watched him write it, I thought about the many poor souls who'd had their diagnosis too late. 'Cure' was no longer an option for them. I was one of the lucky ones, regardless of the hideous list of side effects he'd just rattled off. I was on the right side of this disease. I told myself that I should be very grateful for that. The price to pay for surgery was high. I still felt it was one worth paying.

As the day dragged itself from morning to afternoon, I dozed, on and off, in the coldest room in the world, just next to the nurses' station. The smell of the lunchtime food being delivered to the wards outside my room caused my belly to rumble. A tall nurse entered and for a moment I thought I was getting some food. She quickly dispelled that notion by producing a small, hard plastic pouch with a long neck. The long neck was necessary, as this was the part she told me I had to insert up my bottom. I was to squeeze the contents of the pouch up there and wait for the cramps, spasms and inevitable explosion and evacuation, in preparation for my surgery. She left. I did what I was told. I didn't have to wait long before I was locked in the private bathroom, unable to extricate myself from the cold seat. When I eventually deemed it safe to do so I made my way back to the bed. She reappeared with some pills to take the edge off my nerves. I was then wheeled past 100 flashing ceiling lights and into a lift with some curious visitors who gawped nervously at me. Ten minutes later, I was lying in a holding pen with six others, waiting for our operation slots. When my turn came, I was wheeled into the small room next to the theatre. A very nice anaesthetist talked kindly and cheerily to me as she made three futile attempts to insert a needle into the back of my hand. Her flustered colleague intervened. I counted back from 100, got to 95, and I was gone.

Back in the holding pen, I awoke to someone gently calling my name. Through the fog I could sense that the tennis ball from the biopsy had made its way back up my bottom. My stomach hurt and I was desperate to pee. I was concerned I was going to embarrass myself and wet the bed. I pushed the call button. The nurse was beside my head.

'I need to pee. I think I'm going to wet the bed if I don't get a bedpan quickly.'

She pulled the covers from my leg and detached the bag that was strapped to my ankle, lifting it up so that I could see it. *The day bag! The one that gets connected to the night bag,* was now in her left hand. I thought about singing *Dem Bones* to her but wasn't sure she'd get the joke. She reattached the bag.

'Just let go. You have a catheter fitted. It feels a bit strange at first, but you will get used to it.'

I peeped under the covers. There was a long clear tube poking out of where my penis used to be. She was right. It did feel strange. My urge to pee was fighting a battle with the fear that I would wet myself. The fear of wetting myself was winning at this time and I just couldn't let go of anything. I was still bursting by the time I'd made my way back to the ward. My stomach hurt, my bum hurt, and my catheter was starting to sting. A little tap on the morphine drip did the trick for a while and I slept until Geraldine arrived. She came alone. I didn't want my boys to see me like that. They'd had enough to deal with, what with the whole heart-attack-at-48 thing. I just felt that if they saw me there like that it would cause them distress they didn't need to have. Geraldine held my hand and tried several times to have a conversation with me. The effects of the anaesthetic and morphine meant she spent most of her time watching me sleep and listening to the conversations of the other patients and visitors. I barely remember her leaving but know I felt sad that she had. I hit the drip again. I lowered the bed a little to prepare for what was guaranteed to be a fitful and uncomfortable night. I wasn't wrong.

I opened my eyes and adjusted to the half-light of the ward at night-time. I had no idea what time it was or how long I had slept for since Geraldine had left. What I did know was that I was getting a terrible pain in my stomach and a tugging sensation and stinging in my penis. It took me a moment to fully understand the cause but when my mind cleared, I was aware of a presence sitting on my bed. I looked down to see the covers had been removed. I looked up to see the cause. The top of a young student nurse's head was facing me as she busily fussed about her task. She was oblivious to me. She wasn't aware if I was asleep, awake, comfortable or in agony. She had a job to do, and she was doing it. If she had been more aware, then she would have established that I was most definitely awake and was now in excruciating pain. I could see her hands. They were right next to my shrunken penis. She had her hand on one end of the tube that was resting on my thigh and feeding down the side of the bed and the other hand on the other side of the attachment right next to me. She was muttering to herself as she gave the tube another firm tug. That tug shot a burning pain right up my shrunken shaft and into my bladder, pulling on the inflated balloon which was designed to stop the catheter from being removed from that organ. I shouted out.

'Whoa…Whoa…Whoa…What are you doing?'

I put my hands over hers, to stop her yanking my tube again.

'Oh sorry. I thought you were asleep.'

Thought I was asleep?

'I was asleep, but what you are doing is causing me a bit of pain.'

She stopped momentarily.

'I'm so sorry. I didn't mean to hurt you. It's just I've got to change your catheter and put the night bag on.'

I recognised her mistake, through the haze and the pain.

'Ah, I don't think you are meant to touch that attachment. That stays put for up to a week. The night bag is connected to the day bag down there… if you…'

Before I'd had time to finish the *Dem Bones* conversation, I felt another searing pain shoot up my sorry bits. When I had caught my breath again, I squinted to see her triumphantly holding both ends of the tube she'd been fighting with. Urine dribbled out of each disconnected end and ran onto my legs. She looked at me and at the separated ends. She smiled triumphantly.

'That was a stiff one.'

Oh, the irony.

'All done now, Mr Ferris. I just need to connect the night bag.'

I wanted to tell her again that she was wrong, and she shouldn't have touched that connection. I wanted to let her know that she had hurt me and probably opened me up to a risk of infection. Instead, I said nothing. I watched her, as she beavered away for the next 10 minutes, trying to connect a new bag to the tube coming out of my penis, the tube that she shouldn't have touched in the first place. I had no energy to admonish her. My mind was somewhat preoccupied – all I could concentrate on was the raging fire that she'd started right at the tip of my penis, where the tube entered me. I let her fumble around, until finally she was done. I was relieved to watch her leave. I put the whole episode down to experience and tried to get back to sleep.

The morphine ensured I slept for a while until I was awakened by the sound of metal clanging off a hard surface. I awoke just in time to stop my demented 80-year-old ward-neighbour climbing into my bed beside me. The frame holding the drip he was dragging behind him had clattered off the metal frame of my bed. That was enough to alert the auxiliary nurse, who came racing to the rescue and guided him back to his own bed. But it didn't stop him glaring angrily at me and loudly telling her that I was in his bed. She pulled the curtains around me and told me to watch the TV with my headphones in. It was good advice, but I had to buzz her three times more that night to stop my neighbour clamouring to get in beside me.

On the last occasion I'd buzzed her, the burning sensation at the tip of my penis was so fierce that I swallowed my pride, hid my embarrassment, and asked her if she had anything to take care of the pain. I mentioned the student's efforts earlier and her tug of war with my catheter. She was horrified at the young girl's lack of knowledge of the 'day bag, night bag, don't pull the balloon out of the patient's bladder' procedure, and disappeared to find what she was looking for. She was back in an instant, with a syringe in hand. She pulled the covers off me and sat up on my bed. With the syringe in one hand, she used her finger and thumb on the other to open the tip of my penis, exposing the tube that filled the space in between.

'This will do the trick.'

She inserted the syringe down one side of the tube and then down the other. Each time she felt satisfied with her positioning of it, she gave it a forceful push. Thick clear liquid shot down the sides of the tube and into my penis. The pain was far worse than anything the student nurse had done and caused my eyes to water and I let out a pathetic yelp. But she was right. Within seconds, the anaesthetic was doing its glorious work. She departed, happy with her work and was adamant she'd speak to the student in the morning. I was filled with remorse for complaining and probably getting the poor girl into trouble. I was going to ask her not to speak about it; to let her young friend continue disconnecting the wrong part of the catheter and tugging balloons out of sleeping patient's bladders. Then I thought about the pain I'd been in and the subsequent degradation of having my penis held open while liquid anaesthetic was squirted down inside it. I decided to say nothing.

The student brought me breakfast the next morning. I greedily wolfed down the bread, the vegan spread, and the jam I had asked her for. It was delicious. It was the best vegan spread I had ever tasted. It was so good, I was convinced that it tasted even better than the butter I had given up years earlier. I was filled with remorse about the telling off she'd had or was about to get. I called her over.

'I just wanted to say that was the best vegan spread I have had since giving up dairy products after my heart attack.'

Her face flushed bright red. She looked at the big sign scrawled on the whiteboard behind my bed. VEGAN. She picked up the spread.

'I'm really sorry Mr Ferris. I didn't read the sign. I'm afraid I gave you butter.'

I started to laugh. I could do nothing else. She slipped off and I last saw her talking to the auxiliary nurse, who possessed the expert penis-opening technique. I felt guilty that I had probably got her into trouble. But she definitely needed to learn. For the sake of the hearts and penises of Newcastle, I really hope she did. I never saw her again after that.

CHAPTER 12

Having a drain pulled out of your abdomen is painful and uncomfortable. It's one of those things you don't really think about, and no one really talks about, when you have your surgery. But a day or two after your surgery, a nice nurse comes along and sidles up to you. She smiles and tells you that it will feel a little uncomfortable, and then she firmly tugs the thing though your stomach and out of a hole in your side.

It's the weirdest of sensations having a tube pulled through your insides. My stomach fluttered and cramped as it slid along and out. The nurse puts a little purse against the open hole to catch the residual blood. She told me the doctor would be around in the evening, and with any luck, I could go home in the morning. The thought of going home ensured I was dozing happily again minutes after she'd left.

When I awoke, I could feel a puddle in the bed. The catheter leaking maybe? I pulled the blankets down to see if I could identify the source of the warm wetness that was soaking my sheets. My catheter was intact. My purse wasn't. It had been burst open by the volume of blood that was making its way through the hole in my side where my drain had been. The entire bed was saturated with my blood. I pushed the call button. Ten minutes later I was standing on wobbly legs in front of two or three concerned nurses. Another two were removing the sodden sheets. I wasn't a pretty sight, I'm sure. I swayed there while one nurse lifted my bloodstained gown above my hips. I could see a river of blood running down my side and leg. The catheter poked out of my shrivelled bits, with its half-filled tube, tracing down my other leg. I was grateful for the nurses who stood either side of me. Without their support, my weak legs wouldn't have held me upright long enough for their colleagues to clean up my mess. A busy nurse wiped me down until there were no traces of blood on me. She clipped a fresh purse over the drain hole. A whistling cleaner mopped the thick red puddle of liquid from the floor. Then they were all done. I was relieved when they and the blood had all gone. I lay back in my freshly changed bed.

I had never seen so much of my own blood outside my body before. I wondered if my blood loss would affect my chances of getting home the following day and the thought filled me with dread. I'd had enough of the hospital, the fitful sleep, my poor demented neighbour dragging his catheter all around the ward and trying to climb in beside me, the student nurse and the sick people.

I didn't want to be a sick person, but when you're in hospital, that's what you are. Someone who gets twice daily medications. Someone who's the subject of doctors' rounds. Someone who wears pyjamas and slippers newly bought for the occasion. Someone who gets liquid anaesthetic squirted into his penis. Someone who wakes up in a bed soaked in his own blood. Someone who stands exposed in the middle of a room with a tube dangling from his bits. I didn't want to be that person. I wanted to be me. A healthy person. The person who used to be a professional footballer. The person who loved holidays with my family. The person who loved running up hills and running a company. The person who'd written a manuscript that might one day make him a published author. The person who was a husband, father and now a grandfather. I wanted to be *him*. I wanted to go home. I wanted to lay on my own settee and wish the week away until I could get rid of the catheter and get back to normality. To get back to being me – albeit a new me. A me who no longer had a prostate. That cancerous little walnut was gone. It was now in a lab somewhere, being analysed to establish the extent of the cancer it contained. I would now live my new life without it and the cancer it contained. I just wanted to be out of the hospital, so I could start that life. I was worried the blood loss meant I'd be staying a little longer than I had envisaged. I didn't have too long to fret about it. The following morning's ward round brought me some welcome news.

'You can go home today as planned.'

Dr Alderton's words were unexpected but came as a blessed relief to me. He smiled as the others took notes and looked at the charts that hung on the bottom of my bed. No more sleepless nights protecting my territory from the catheter-dragger. The previous night had been the worst yet. The poor confused man had spent the whole night calling for his wife, and marching up and down the dimly lit, nurse-less corridors, all the while, dragging and clanking the long metal pole that held his drip or his catheter. When he wasn't doing that, he was still fighting me for my bed. I'd tried on several occasions to gently point him in the direction of his own bed, but it was a constant battle. It was a battle I had nearly lost on one occasion. Despite fighting hard to stay awake, I had slipped into a light sleep, only to be stirred by my blankets being pulled back and his bony bum pushing against my side as he fought hard to get in beside me. In the end, I had sat upright and stayed awake all night, too frightened to sleep, for fear that I would wake up with him snuggled up next to me.

It was the evening by the time I got home. I was in a lot of pain, but I was glad to be out of the hospital. Geraldine did a better job than the student nurse and connected my night bag to the day bag. I settled down for a good night's sleep in my own bed. That was until the first spasm in my bladder had me gasping for breath. It was followed by another, then another. It was excruciating. By the time the spasms had passed, the sweat that was running down my brow was mingling with the tears that were streaming down my cheeks. It's almost impossible to convey the level of pain I experienced that first night at home, as the spasms caused by my bladder trying to expel the balloon of the catheter had me bent double and screeching in agony. When daylight came, I made my way wearily to the settee and tried to find a comfortable position to sleep. Some strong painkillers ensured I made up for the restless night that had just passed. When I opened my eyes, I felt my mouth go dry before watery bile filled it. I swallowed hard to stop myself from vomiting over the duvet I was wrapped in.

'Do you want something to eat?'

Geraldine had made her way from the kitchen, with her plates of food, and sat down on the chair opposite me. The smell wafting from her plate, ensured the contents of my stomach found their resting place on the duvet at the second attempt. Geraldine rolled up the liquid- filled duvet, removed it, and cleaned me up. The foul-smelling food was still in the room. I felt my mouth watering again.

'You'll have to take that into the kitchen and close the door. It's making me feel really sick. I don't want anything to eat. I don't think I could keep it down.'

When she'd left the room, the nausea subsided. But the relief was only temporary. When she came back a little later and kissed my head, the smell of her perfume had me retching again. If it wasn't her food, it was her perfume. If it wasn't her perfume, it was her hair. If it wasn't her hair, it was her breath. I was so nauseous that I had to ask her to stay away from me.

'I think I'm allergic to you!'

'Thanks!'

'I'm serious. I can't stand your smell. It makes me feel really sick.'

She laughed.

'You have such a charming way with words. I can't change my smell! Do you think we should call the doctor and tell him you are not eating, and everything is making you nauseous? Maybe it's the medication?'

She had a point. I'd come out of hospital with a cocktail of medication including an injection I had to administer into my thigh every day. Maybe those, on top of my heart medication, were the cause of my problems. One totally pointless telephone conversation with an on-call GP later, and we were none the wiser. She was very polite on the phone, but also dismissive. She said it was just a natural reaction to the surgery, and I was due at the hospital again in less than a week to have my catheter removed, so could discuss it again then. Meanwhile I should drink plenty and eat when I could.

The days dragged and the nights were restless. My sisters, Elizabeth and Denise, came to see me. They travelled from Ireland to look after me for a night, as Geraldine had to drive Ciaran to Manchester. It was a Saturday. I was due to have my catheter removed on the Monday. They were a little shocked by my appearance. Five days of not eating or sleeping had obviously taken its toll. I spent the day sleeping on the settee, ignoring my caring and concerned sisters. To my great embarrassment, Denise had to help me upstairs and put me into bed. Once there, I lay freezing and shivering as she wrapped the quilt around me and connected the night bag to the day bag. Geraldine got back in the early hours. Her warmth next to me ensured I finally got some sleep. I was glad I had my back to her so I couldn't smell her.

*   *   *

Monday arrived. I could barely walk the distance from the car to the hospital on the morning my catheter was to be removed. I stood at the reception, holding on to Geraldine for support. The nurse directed us to a chair, to wait our turn. There were two men opposite us. They were laughing and joking and looked like they hadn't a care in the world. They could very easily have been mistaken for visitors, if it wasn't for the give-away catheter bags that poked out from below their trousers. My hand was ice cold and shaking when I slipped it into Geraldine's. I nudged her.

'There's something not right here. Those two are here to get their catheters out, but they look great and don't seem to be in any discomfort. I feel like a complete bag of shit.'

She squeezed my hand.

'You're here now in the right place. Maybe when they take the catheter out, you'll feel better.'

The nurse poked her head around the door and ushered us into her small office. I told her about not feeling well, not eating and being allergic to my wife. She asked me if I had brought some tight-fitting underwear. I chastised myself for not reading the instructions properly and told her I only had boxer shorts. She produced a pair of net-like pants with a pad inside that looked like a Dr White's sanitary towel from the 1970s. In fact, the last time I'd seen a Dr White's, was *in* the 1970s. I'd found my mother's stash in the twin-tub washing machine and was fascinated as to why my new doctors' mask only had a loop at one end and a long piece of string on the other. I was expertly wrapping the long string around my ear when my mother came into the kitchen. She snatched it off me with one hand and clipped me around the offending ear with the other.

The nurse's voice brought me back to this decade. We had a brief conversation about erectile dysfunction. She followed that up by producing two packs of sildenafil. *That's Viagra for those of us in the know.* Apparently, because Dr Alderton had spared the nerves to my penis during surgery, I might get natural erections again sometime in the next 18 months, but the likelihood was that I would need a little help from the tablets as well. While she was talking, she ushered me onto the bed in the corner of her room and asked me to remove my clothing. She slipped the net pants with the Dr White's inside up my legs in preparation.

'Could you just cough gently for me?'

As I did what I was told, she deflated the balloon and pulled it out of my bladder, through my urethra, and out of the end of my stinging penis. It wasn't too painful. It was just sickeningly alien. Having the drain tube pulled through my stomach a week before was bad enough, but a deflated balloon being sucked out of the bladder and urethra was infinitely more unpleasant. She expertly slipped my net pants up and over my exposed bits, but not before I'd had time to look down and assess the sorry state of my shrivelled, stinging mess of penis.

'If you could go back to the waiting room and drink three cups of water, we just need to see that everything is working as it should be, before we let you home.'

I was unsteady on my feet as I left the room. I held on to Geraldine's arm as she guided me back to the chair. I was glad to be rid of the catheter. No more spasms in the night, or the need for Geraldine to squirt anaesthetic into my willy. I didn't have the energy to walk to the water fountain, so Geraldine brought me my water. I drank my three cups. When I felt the need to pee, I made my way into the toilet. My head was spinning a little as I stood over the toilet. I held the measuring jug and waited. The first drops came out blood red. I looked down into the jug and could see the red turning to clear liquid as the urine diluted the blood. Everything was working as it should. My reattached tubes connecting my bladder and urethra were intact. All was good in the world... except it wasn't. The jug I was holding started to spin in one direction, and the toilet bowl below spun the other way. I felt my legs turn to jelly. The colours in the room faded. *I was going and I knew I was going.* I tried to sit down on the cold floor, in the hope that by doing so, I could somehow stop whatever was coming. I managed to get the jug onto the floor. Then everything turned to black.

When I came around, I was lying on my back on the toilet floor. My head was jammed up against the door. I could hear the sounds of the waiting room on the other side of it, but I couldn't move, or call out. I knew Geraldine was sitting five feet away from me, yet oblivious to my predicament. I don't know how long I'd laid there but I stayed a bit longer until I felt able to get up off the floor. I pulled myself up using the door handle and managed to open the door. Geraldine's face was white as I approached her. She rushed from her seat to greet me.

'Jesus. You look awful. Are you alright?'

I took her hand for support and shook my head.

'I think I fainted.'

Geraldine shouted for the nurse. She took hold of my other hand and guided me back to her office. Ten minutes later Dr Alderton was holding my hand. I told him about the week I'd had; the nausea, the spasms, the lack of eating and sleeping. He made a call to the ward. An hour later I was back in the same place I had left behind last week. This time I would stay there until they could work out exactly what was wrong with me.

CHAPTER 13

I don't believe I have ever felt as ill as I did that day. If I have, I don't remember it. I lay in the bed while several doctors and nurses scurried around me. One took blood, one set up a drip, one checked my temperature and took my blood pressure, while another booked X-rays and scans. The flurry of activity was subsiding when a tiny Sri Lankan doctor popped his head around the corner of my closed curtain. He was very pleasant as he took hold of my hand. He rubbed my freezing hand furiously between his, before slapping it hard several times.

'You are very white. Very white.'

I mustered a whisper.

'I'm Irish. My natural colour is a bluish-white.'

I don't think he was ready for the attempt at humour from his sick patient. Either that or my effort just wasn't that funny. He slapped me again. He shook his head. He was mumbling to himself as he was making his exit.

'Very white. Very white. Very white.'

The frenzied activity gave way to two hours of boredom as the daylight faded into early night. Geraldine shuffled uncomfortably in her chair and I dribbled uncontrollably into my Dr White. No matter how hard I tried to stop it, I just couldn't interrupt the steady stream of urine seeping from me onto my saturated pad. The realisation of what that meant for me, only added to the misery of what was already a bad day. I turned to Geraldine and disturbed her efforts to sleep.

'I'm incontinent. I'm fucking incontinent. For fuck's sake!'

She took my hand and leaned over the bed.

'It's alright. The doctor told you this might happen, remember? He said it might only be temporary.'

I wasn't in the mood for her calm reassurance. I snapped at her.

'Ah, OK. That's alright then. I'm only pissing myself temporarily then. No worries there. Might last a month, a year or a lifetime, but it will all be good in the end. I must remember to stop complaining.'

She rubbed my hand and ignored my tone.

'I'm not saying it's OK. It's far from it. It's pretty shit, but for the minute, it's the least of your worries. You haven't been well since the surgery. You fainted this morning and you look like death warmed up. Let's deal with what's in front of us today and worry about the other stuff when we get this sorted.'

I squeezed her hand.

'Sorry, I'm just fed up. Fed up and scared. Scared of what's happening to me now and scared of the changes from the surgery that I can't undo.'

She sat back on her uncomfortable chair.

'Whatever changes the surgery has caused is better than the alternative. You could be wandering around with cancer growing inside of you and be none the wiser. We are lucky. We found it in time for them to cut it out. Whatever the surgery has done, I don't care, I just want you here for me and the boys.'

I looked at her face. It was the most familiar face in the world to me. One I had looked into since it was 13 years old. She was 50 now, and still as beautiful to me as she was when I had first set eyes on her. What dreams we'd shared, what hopes we'd cherished and what fears we'd faced. But in the last three years everything had started to crumble. My heart attack and now this. She had faced them all with quiet stoicism and courage. She'd supported me unwaveringly and held our family together through it all. But when I looked at her there in that dark hospital ward, she looked tired. No. It was more than that. It was more than just tiredness. She looked frightened. I felt a rush of guilt that I had brought all of this to her door. I pushed the button to raise my bed, so that I was sitting up next to her.

'I love you very much. You know that, right?'

She smiled wearily.

'I love you too.'

'No, I mean whatever happens, I need you to know that I have always loved you. Even if I'm gone, I want you to know that I couldn't have loved you more.'

She shook her head.

'Don't talk like that. They will be in here in a minute and get to the bottom of what's going on. Then we will be home in a day or two and can put this behind us.'

I hadn't meant to be so morbid but I had never felt so weak. I had never felt so sick. I was getting worse by the hour. I felt like I was dying. Whatever was causing me to feel so ill needed to be dealt with and dealt with quickly.

Hours passed before a porter came. He lifted me into a wheelchair and took me to get some chest X-rays. He left us in the waiting room of the X-ray department. There was no one around and we sat in silence. Geraldine tried on several occasions to make small talk, but I didn't have the energy or inclination to respond. I was unaware of the time or the day now. Maybe it was eight or maybe it was nine. I had no idea and I didn't care. My hands were shaking, my mouth was dry and my head was pounding. Someone brought me through for the X-ray. She asked me to stand up and put my chest against a whiteboard. I tried to get up from my wheelchair, but my legs weren't responding to my feeble commands. When I had failed to stand at the third attempt, the radiographer helped me out of the chair. On vibrating legs, I held on to the X-ray machine. I hung on there for minutes, but it felt like forever. I was relieved when she detached my grip and slumped me back in the chair. I don't remember how we got back to the ward that night, or how I ended up in bed. I was lost, off in another world. No longer part of this one. I was still vaguely aware of Geraldine's presence beside me, but I was no longer capable of communicating with her. Something was desperately wrong. I knew that much. Someone touched my arm and stirred me from my slumber. I tried to focus through the fog. I could see Dr Alderton leaning over me. He was talking to me.

'You are not a well man, Paul. Your tests have come back. I'm afraid you have sepsis and anaemia. We are going to administer some intravenous antibiotics for the sepsis, and you will also need a blood transfusion for the anaemia. Do you understand?' I didn't – but nodded in agreement. I drifted off to sleep and only awoke again in the middle of the night when the nurse came to administer my latest dose of antibiotics. She was gone and I drifted away again. The next time I surfaced, was when the lights flickered into life on the ward and the trolley serving breakfasts competed with the one serving tablets.

'Good morning, Paul. How are you today?'

I looked up to see a bearded junior doctor at the foot of my bed. I heard him clearly and I saw him clearly. It was like the dark tunnel I had been travelling down had suddenly given way to brilliant sunshine. The nausea had gone completely. The smell of the toast on the breakfast trolley wasn't making me retch. I don't know whether it was the regular doses of antibiotics, or the two pints of some kind stranger's blood I couldn't even remember receiving that had done the trick, but something had. That morning, I didn't know and I didn't care. I by no means felt well, but compared to how I had felt just a few hours before it was like a miracle had happened. I wouldn't have thought it possible to go from my sick place to my new place so rapidly. I smiled at the doctor.

'I am feeling much better. Do you think I could go home today?'

He shook his head and laughed loudly at the ridiculousness of my question.

'Dr Alderton will be around after his surgery today and you can speak to him about that. But you have been very sick, and I don't think you will be going home for a day or two just yet.'

Defeated on the stupid question, I looked for victory elsewhere.

'Would I be able to have some toast?'

That was a much more sensible question for him.

'You can have as much toast as you like, Mr Ferris. It is good to see you looking so well and clearly feeling much better.'

I really was feeling much better. I had four slices of thin white toast with spread and jam. It tasted better than the best meal at the best restaurant I had ever eaten in. I only stopped when my stomach started to hurt, otherwise I'd have eaten the whole loaf. I was still contemplating my miracle recovery when I reached for my phone to text Geraldine the good news. The screen flickered into life. Twenty-five unread emails. I wanted to ignore them but I've never been able to do that. So I scrolled down. There were 18 from work, one from my friend Peter, five junk mails and one from Guy Rose. I searched around for my glasses. We'd forgotten to bring them yesterday. We didn't know I'd be staying. I clicked on his email and made the screen as big as I could. I had to read it twice to make sure my eyes weren't playing tricks on me. They weren't. What was on front of me was the second miracle that had occurred in my life yesterday. Guy, the literary agent, who I'd never met or even spoken to, was very excited to report that he'd secured me a publisher for my manuscript. Not only that, he had secured Hodder and Stoughton, part of the Hachette Group, and one of the biggest publishers in the world! Well, he hadn't exactly secured Hodder yet. He'd had a very positive response from a representative of Hodder. Not just any representative though. Roddy Bloomfield, the editor of over 1,000 sports books and undoubtedly the most respected practitioner in his field, had read my manuscript and was interested in making an advance offer for it.

Advance offer! I lay back in the bed. How strange this life is that we live? I don't think I have ever had a darker day than the one I had the day I received Guy's email. Sepsis and anaemia, antibiotics and blood transfusions, sickness and confusion. That was my day. The week before had been an ugly one. The surgery, the spasms, the sleepless nights. The sickness, weakness, injections and catheter. It had all left me dejected, disillusioned and feeling overwhelmed by the turn my life had taken. But now this, right in the middle of my darkest moment, right in the middle of the mess of yesterday, a literary agent and a book editor were in early communication with each other to see if they could strike a deal to publish my memoir. I would have paid Hodder to publish it. Never mind negotiate an advance for it. I looked around the ward. There were sick people everywhere. I was one of them. Yet, I suddenly felt alive. I wanted to shout across the room to anyone who would listen. Tell them I was going to be a published author. Me, from St Patrick's secondary school in Lisburn, failed footballer, was going to be a published author! I tried to think of another footballer who had done that. I don't mean have a ghost-written book published. There were hundreds who'd done that. I mean have a book published they'd actually written themselves. I couldn't. I couldn't think of a single one. *To hell with the heart attack. Fuck prostate cancer. Bollox to sepsis and anaemia. I was going to be a published author!* I felt like I was floating above the bed. Even the spurts of urine that were soaking my already sodden pad couldn't bring me back down to earth.

I stayed in the hospital for three more torturous nights. I don't think I slept more than three hours a night. I defy anyone to do better than that in a hospital ward. The noises at night, the light and the patients roaming the corridors. Why are there are always patients roaming the corridors? All of it conspires to rob you of any kind of rest. But I didn't care. I had something to hang on to, something to focus on, and something to look forward to. I'd got rid of my cancer, my catheter, my sepsis and my anaemia. Now I had a book deal coming my way. This life wasn't so bad after all.

I monitored the negotiations from afar. I was exhilarated when I could finally see them reaching the point of agreement. They gently nudged and pushed back, and nudged again, until they settled on an agreed advance for my manuscript. Guy emailed me to say he thought it was worth more but hadn't wanted to push it too hard on this occasion. *I really didn't care.* Any offer seemed like a pretty good offer to me, for something I'd tapped out on two fingers at the kitchen table. I was so excited, that as soon as I signed the contract, I bought a frame and placed the agreement in it. I hung it in my living room so that I could look at it every day. Apart from the heart disease and cancer, I felt that life couldn't really get much better for me in the circumstances. Then it did.

I was lying on my settee watching some ancient midday matinee when I received an email from a production company in London. They had read *An Irish Heartbeat*, my self-published novel from five years previously. They'd loved it and were wondering if anyone had secured film rights options on it? I nearly fell off the settee. I told them no one had taken the film rights option. In truth, no one had even read the bloody thing. Never mind take the film rights option on it. They said they wanted the option. I told them they could most certainly have it. They sent a contract. I signed it. Then I bought another frame to put it in.

I was so high with it all that I almost forgot about the cancer. Almost. I checked my diary. I needed a blood test to see if all the cancer had been removed through surgery. I had an appointment booked for the following week with Dr Alderton, where I would find out the results of the blood test and the pathology of my cancerous prostate. That reality wasn't quite enough to bring my feet back to the ground. It did, however, niggle at the back of my mind, even among all of the euphoria of book deals and film rights. None of those things would mean anything if I didn't have good health to experience them. I booked my blood tests and waited for my appointment. Hopefully all would be well.

CHAPTER 14

It's hard to explain the stress I felt when I was sitting in a hospital waiting room knowing that the overworked doctor I was waiting patiently to see could drop a bomb straight into the middle of my busy life. Yes, I'd taken the decision to have my prostate removed, so that the cancer would be cut out for good. Then I could become someone who once had cancer. I would be one of the lucky ones who'd caught it early and snuffed it out, before it had the chance to do the same to me.

I had had my 'bloods' taken at the GP surgery a few days before my appointment with the urologist. I could have called the reception there and asked for the results. I knew what represented good ones and not so good ones. Good results, after the removal of a cancerous prostate, are PSA levels of less than 0.03, the minimum measurable amount. But I didn't call the GP surgery in case the person reading them to me over the phone gave me bad news. That would have sent me into a tailspin for days while I waited for my urology appointment. So I now sat nervously waiting for my name to be called.

Dr Alderton smiled as I entered his room. I took that as a good sign.

'Good to see you again Mr Ferris. You are certainly looking a lot better than the last time I saw you. How have you been feeling?'

I gave him chapter and verse on my incontinence and my erectile dysfunction. I was still wetting myself into the pads I had discreetly purchased online. Don't get me wrong, I wasn't pouring pints of urine into them, just dribbles every now and then, but too often for my liking and my self-esteem though. There is something very disconcerting about casually chatting with a friend or a work colleague while all the while you are simultaneously wetting yourself. Or being out for dinner in a nice restaurant and ordering your meal while urine seeps out of you under the table. Everything on the surface appears the same. But it's not the same. It's stomach churning to know you have no control of such a basic function. I told Dr Alderton I was using two light pads a day. It was a vast improvement from the four heavy ones I had started out with. I was doing my pelvic floor exercises religiously and they seemed to be helping matters. To my great relief, he felt that I was on my way to becoming continent again at some unspecified time in the future.

The erectile dysfunction was a more complex matter. Since the surgery and having the catheter removed, I hadn't had so much as a flicker of life in that department. In fact, what I had been left with was a leathery, wet, shrunken mess. Not really what any man wants between his legs. Or any woman for that matter! I had taken the Viagra as prescribed, but the only part of my body it had affected was my head. It had given me an intolerable headache and a crimson-red face. We had a lengthy discussion on my continued ability to have an orgasm without an erection. I told him they weren't what they were cracked up to be. We explored the possibility of a penis pump. It was some sort of vacuum device that I would slip my bits into. I'd seal it, then pump my reluctant willy back to life. Once it had responded I would quickly snap a ring around the base of it. This would, in turn, trap just enough blood to enable me to have a stuffable erection. *What the fuck was a stuffable erection?*

Whatever it was, I didn't fancy one. I'm not sure anybody would. I was happy to persevere with a different form of medication, an alternative to Viagra. Hopefully this one would affect my nether regions rather than my head. I'd wait for the nerves, that he assured me were still intact, to spark spontaneously and miraculously back into life someday in the future. Then I would be back to normal. Not normal exactly. An orgasm without producing semen is never normal. An orgasm without a prostate is nothing like an orgasm with one. An orgasm minus an erection… well, that seems just wrong.

When we'd finished discussing my erectile dysfunction, we moved on to a debate about the appropriateness of the term itself when used to describe the predicament I, and many other men, found ourselves in after surgery. I already deeply resented it. One minute, I was perfectly intact and functioning very well down there. The next, I'm a sufferer of erectile dysfunction. I told him it would be much more accurate to call it 'surgically induced erectile dysfunction.' It just sounded better to me. No disrespect to Dr Alderton, and all the other brilliant surgeons out there performing textbook prostatectomies, but when you are on the other side of the knife, and trying to cope with life afterwards, you can't help feeling butchered, mutilated even. Erections, and the ability to spontaneously generate them, go right to the heart of what makes a man a man. Having that ability cut out of you, even though you know it's for the best and the alternative is unthinkable, doesn't make the pain of losing the life you once had any easier to bear.

When we had finished discussing my philosophical objections to the medical terminology used to describe where I now found myself in life, we got down to discussing the results of the surgery and the pathology of my recently removed cancerous prostate.

'Your PSA is undetectable Mr Ferris. Less than 0.03. That is really great news at this stage and is exactly what I would want to see.'

I felt a little rush of adrenalin.

'That's great news and makes the decision to have the surgery feel worthwhile.'

I was still digesting the good news, when he moved on to the pathology of my diseased prostate itself.

'There was a very high volume of cancer and it was in both lobes of your prostate. I have no doubt that it would have impacted on your life had it remained undetected.'

More good news.

'Just as well I had it removed then. I'm really happy with that decision now.'

He moved quickly on to grading the cancer that was found in the lab. Mine had a Gleason score of 7. This was made up of a combination of two numbers. In my case, the majority of the cancer was 3. This, apparently, was a good thing. The higher the number the more aggressive and severe the cancer was. So 5 and 5, with a total of 10, wouldn't be too good at all; 3 and 4, equalling 7, was better than 4 and 3, equalling 7, as that would have meant the cancer was more aggressive or more advanced. Anyway, lots of number combinations that I didn't really understand were for him to worry about. And he didn't seem too worried at all.

He moved onto the 'margins' now. All this new language was something I had to familiarise myself with. Margins are very important where cancer is concerned. Negative margins are the holy grail and the goal of surgery. Cancer contained. Cancer cut out. Cancer cured. *Merry Christmas one and all!*

'Your margins were all clear.'

The good news kept on coming.

'Apart from a tiny positive margin at the apical margin of the prostate.'

It's amazing how a mood can change in an instant. I felt my stomach turn a little as he'd uttered the words.

'That's not good, right? That means some cancer was left behind?'

He smiled reassuringly.

'Not necessarily in this case. The prostate doesn't have a defined border at that point where your positive margin is. It is such a small positive margin and it's Gleason 3 (those numbers again) at the margin. It may well be, that during your surgery, I have cut through the cancerous cells and killed them off anyway. The most important thing is that your PSA is currently undetectable. We will just keep an eye on you every three months. If there is no change, then all well and good. If it rises, we have the option of salvage radiotherapy.

Salvage radiotherapy?

I didn't like the sound of that. Cue another philosophical debate about the medical terminology in use around prostate cancer. 'Salvage' made me think of one thing only – wreckage. To me, salvage meant trying to rescue something that was already a lost cause. *Get what you can before the whole thing is beyond all repair.* He agreed the terminology could be better, but insisted that even if the PSA started to rise that I wasn't a lost cause. The positive margin wasn't ideal, but he would be much more concerned if it was accompanied by an elevated PSA.

I left his office dazed but reassured. I'd chosen the nuclear option of having my prostate removed. That was supposed to be the end of my cancer journey. Now, I realised it was potentially only the beginning. That thought filled me with dread. His calm demeanour had tempered my fear a little and I was relatively calm about it all. Then I went home and spent the next three hours on the internet. I searched medical terms like positive margins, salvage radiotherapy, rising PSA. I also looked at several other things any sensible person of sound mind and judgement would avoid at all costs. By the time I'd closed my laptop, I had convinced myself that my surgery had failed. I was certain that the nine-month gap between my visit to the GP and eventual surgery had been potentially fatal. That time lag was surely the difference between a high volume of cancer and a low volume of cancer. Time enough for a clear margin to become a positive margin. My surgery had left me walking around pissing my pants, erection-less and semen-less. Not to mention it had also led to sepsis and anaemia. Now, here I was on a three-monthly clock waiting to find out if it had been any kind of success at all. If my PSA levels were to rise again, then as far as I was concerned it had all been for nothing. That thought was gut punching.

To take my mind off my troubles I booked a trip for me and Geraldine to go to Killarney, in the west of Ireland. It was only for two days, but just getting on a plane, arriving at the hotel and being in Ireland lifted my spirits. We got up on our first morning and walked for hours through the beautiful Gap of Dunloe. We'd been there with the kids on a summer holiday years before and I'd loved it. As we walked through this green mountainous paradise, I was back there again with them. They were running, laughing, throwing pebbles into the lake, gorging on their picnic. Their excited laughter echoing off the hills.

As I breathed the crisp air into my lungs, the weight of the world lifted from my shoulders. We had dinner in a beautiful restaurant in the town. We drank Guinness. We listened to a live band in one bar before heading to the next, and repeated the process until the music stopped and we could drink no more. We held on to each other as we started to make our way back to the hotel. We needed to, otherwise one or both of us would have fallen over from the effects of too much of Arthur's finest. It was the happiest I'd felt since my cancer diagnosis and certainly since the whole positive margin, salvage radiotherapy conversation. Life felt good again. Nothing had changed. Geraldine was laughing beside me and linking her arm in mine. Granted it was only to stop herself from falling over, but she was holding my arm just the same. We were in Ireland, where I always loved to be. We were drunk and carefree. All was well in our world. Nothing could spoil that moment... *except*. Except the little spurt of piss that hit my light pad as I took the first steps up the hill towards the hotel. It was followed by another, then another, and yet another. By the time the hotel came into view, I was pissing like a fountain with every step I took. The pad had surrendered 20 paces back and my jeans were now being soaked with every stride. Where are Billy Connolly's incontinence pants when you need them? I'd cried with laugher when I'd watched that sketch as a young man. It didn't seem so funny now. When I reached the sanctuary of the hotel bedroom, I closed the bathroom door. I pulled off my sticky jeans and surveyed the wet mess. I slid down the door. My anger, frustration and embarrassment ran down my cheeks.

How could I possibly hope to function at work, or have a normal social life, if I couldn't walk from the pub to the hotel without tying two knots round my ankles to stem the tide that gushed out of me and ran down my legs? I felt like one of those strange kids' dolls you see advertised at Christmas, where you pour liquid in one end and it pees it out the other as quickly as it went in. Geraldine knocked on the door.

'You alright?'

I pulled myself together.

'Yes. All good. Just had a bit of a problem with my pad. I can't hold my drink anymore.'

I opened the door and held up my soaked jeans.

'Literally!'

No matter how long you've known your partner or how much intimacy you've shared in the past, it's fucking humiliating to be standing in front of that person holding a pair of piss-soaked jeans in the air. Being drunk when you are doing so helps a little, but it doesn't entirely rid you of the shame. Geraldine took them from me.

'Oh God. They're soaked through. Did you bring another pair with you?'

That snapped me out of my self-pity.

'Shit. I didn't. Cos we were flying on Ryanair, and they charge you for breathing, I only packed these.'

Washing your piss-stained jeans in the hotel sink, while your wife lies patiently in bed waiting for you to finish, puts a bit of a dampener on any romantic break you think you're having. Killarney doesn't feel as pretty when you are visiting the sights in jeans that didn't quite dry well enough on the radiator overnight.

Two nights of taking my medication an hour before bed in the vain hope it would somehow spark my reluctant penis back to life meant that by the end of the trip I was less relaxed than I had been at the start of it. There was so little sign of life down there that I actually started dreaming of the success I might have had with the vacuum pump. If only I had accepted the doctor's offer to refer me for a fitting before our trip. I could have just disappeared into the bathroom, run the taps to hide the sound of the inflation, and deftly pumped my recalcitrant friend back to life. Geraldine could have lay in bed unaware that at any minute I would burst through the door, stuffable erection at the ready. No problem that it had to be held aloft by two rings strangling the life out of the dormant little bastard.

CHAPTER 15

Cancer is everywhere when you have cancer. You can't avoid it, no matter how hard you try. It appears on every ad break on the TV. One minute you're happily sipping a glass of wine watching your favourite ITV drama, and the next there is some poor soul with no hair staring out of the screen at you. Or even worse, it's some innocent child who hasn't had a chance to live before having to deal with the ramifications of a life-changing or life-ending diagnosis. The radio is no better. You can be humming along to Van Morrison or whoever else takes your fancy. You're just idling your time away in the latest traffic jam you're trapped in. Before you know it *Brown Eyed Girl* is being followed by a very stern man, who solemnly asks you if you know that prostate cancer kills one man every 45 seconds in the UK. *Every 45 seconds. In the UK!*

Maybe the UK is the problem? *It's deadly living here.* I'm going to move to someplace where prostate cancer doesn't kill me every 45 seconds. Every 45 months sounds better. Every 45 years; now you are really talking.

I know these ads are necessary. I know they serve a great purpose in raising awareness and generating much-needed funds for research, but those ads made for some uncomfortable moments with my children. Having spent months telling them I was going to be alright, those ads would come on, and the awkward questions would start. Ciaran shared the car with me on his school run. Every day, there was sure to be a cancer advert, or a story in the news of a cancer tragedy. I'd quickly switch the station or look to see if he had his headphones on. Most days he'd be listening to some American from the 'hood', educating him on bitches, blades and whatever else they could swear into his not-from-the-hood ears. On one occasion, I was too slow to change the station and he was having a break from his music.

'That doesn't sound too good dad. That doesn't mean you, does it?'

I was annoyed at myself for not getting the prostate cancer advert off the radio in time.

'What?'

'One man dies from prostate cancer every 45 seconds in the UK. That doesn't sound great to me. Does that mean you are going to die from it?'

'What? Me? Of course not. Don't be daft. I'm fine.'

Well, as fine as I can be pissing into a pad and with no prospect of an erection on the horizon anytime soon son, but that's not a conversation either of us would wish to have... ever.

'The surgeon removed my prostate, and my PSA is undetectable. As long as everything stays like that, then I'm going to be fine. Those adverts are referring to men who don't get checked in time and the cancer has already spread. It's very sad. Luckily, I got checked in time and had the cancer removed.'

That should have been enough for him, but it wasn't.

'But you didn't get it all removed, did you? I heard you talking to mum the other night about the positive margin. A positive margin means there was cancer left behind, right? So all of the cancer has not gone, has it?'

He definitely had me there.

'Technically that is correct, but in my case the surgeon said he probably killed off any cancerous cells when he cut through the tissue to remove my prostate. Besides, it's all about my bloods and my bloods three months after surgery were perfect. Less than 0.03 – and that means cancer is undetectable in my body. PSA only registers if there are prostate cells there, good or cancerous. In my case it is completely undetectable.'

He wasn't convinced.

'You say that, but I heard you telling mum you were worried about the positive margin.'

'When did you hear that?'

'I was in the kitchen on Friday night and you were talking about it in the living room. If you are not alright, I would rather know that, than you tell me everything is fine.'

Did you know that prostate cancer kills one man every 45 seconds in the UK?

Those fucking adverts! Another one had come on as I was trying to reassure my 16-year-old son.

I turned the radio off.

'Listen son. If we were talking on Friday night, we were probably drinking wine, too. Don't pay attention to our ramblings. I'm fine and I will be fine. Please don't worry.'

'Are you sure?'

'Yes, I'm sure.'

He seemed satisfied though I wasn't sure I had totally convinced him. Or myself. He put his headphones on and I lost him again to Ty Dolla Sign.

He'd had a point on the positive margin stuff. I'm a natural born worrier. Ever since it had been mentioned to me it had played on my mind. Not every day, not all the time. Just most days, most of the time. A positive margin to me meant that my surgery and my battles with sepsis and anaemia might all have been rendered pointless. My lack of erections, my missing semen, and my saturated jeans had all been indignities I hadn't needed to suffer. Yet the reality was that my PSA was the key. For the moment it was completely undetectable. That was a reason to be cheerful. If it stayed that way, I was home – if not quite dry.

The ongoing worry over the positive margin ensured that I called my GP practice for the results of my latest PSA test results in advance of my three-monthly follow-up with Dr Alderton. I had toyed with the idea of leaving it until I was sitting in front of him, but I was worried about my reaction or ability to rationalise matters if the PSA had risen. So instead, I called the GP. I wanted advance notice of the results. Half-way through my phone conversation with the impatient receptionist I wished I hadn't bothered.

'Your bloods have come back perfect Mr Ferris. Thank you. Bye.'

'Wait. Wait. Before you go. Could you please tell me the actual results?'

I got to her just before she cut me off.

'Yes. They are perfect. As I said. Thank you.'

She was on her way again.

'No. No. I appreciate they are perfect. Could you just tell me the actual reading on your screen please?'

I listened to her loud sigh as she frantically tapped on a keyboard.

'Ah yes. Here it is. Your PSA is 0.3 and the doctor is happy with that.'

0.3!

My heart started thumping and my head followed suit.

'Sorry. Could you please read that again for me? You said 0.3?'

Another loud sigh.

'Yes, that's right. 0.3.'

I could hear the tremble in my voice.

'But that's not good. It should be 0.03 not 0.3, 0.3 means it's 10 times worse than my first test and my PSA is detectable again. I don't understand why the doctor would be happy with that?'

My thumping chest almost drowned out her final sigh.

'It says on here 0.3. Oh wait. It says 0.03. I'm so sorry. I missed out a decimal place.'

It was my turn to sigh. I wanted to hear her say it again. I didn't care if I was holding her day to ransom.

'Thank you. Can you just confirm for me one more time please? What exactly does it say on your screen?'

'Certainly Mr Ferris. I can confirm your blood results are PSA 0.03 and the doctor is happy with them.'

The relief when I hung up quickly gave way to euphoria. After my conversation with Ciaran in the car and all of my worrying, the busy receptionist had initially floored me with her erroneous reading of my results. For a fleeting moment she'd had me believe that my PSA had climbed tenfold within three months. It had filled me with complete horror. For those few moments my biggest fears had become my reality. I thought that my surgery had failed, and I was on my way to salvage radiotherapy to try and rescue the wreckage. But I wasn't. I was on my way to getting rid of my cancer.

The call to the GP did have one benefit. Later, as I sat in the hospital, waiting to be called into Dr Alderton's office, I at least knew that he would only have good news for me. I'd had my blood test results and they were 0.03. They were perfect. I knew what he would have to say before I even entered his room.

Good news Mr Ferris. Bloods are perfect. No change. Don't worry about the positive margin. Sorry to hear about the incontinence and lack of erections. See you in three months.

I made my way along the corridor, entered his office and sat triumphantly in the same chair I'd sat in when he'd dropped the cancer bomb on me.

'How have you been generally over the past three months Mr Ferris?'

Dr Alderton greeted me politely and sat down in front of his desk. Over his shoulder, Julie smiled at me, from her perch on his treatment couch.

'I would say I've been pretty good, lack of erections and wetting myself apart. I'm a bit fragile mentally with it all, but I guess that's to be expected. In the main I'd say I'm making good progress. I'm back at work three days a week and trying to get some normality back really.'

He probably only wanted a quick 'I'm doing well' but I have a tendency to talk too much, especially when I'm nervous. It's impossible not to be nervous when you are in a consultant's office talking about cancer, even if you know that your bloods are perfect and that you haven't got cancer anymore.

Dr Alderton scrolled down the screen in front of him until he found what he was looking for.

'I presume you've seen your latest blood results?'

He turned the monitor to face me.

'I have. I gather I'm doing very well. It's good that they haven't changed, and my PSA is still undetectable. I was a bit concerned with the positive margin stuff at our last appointment, but the latest negative blood result on top of the first one has given me a little more confidence.'

I was talking too much again. He found the perfect words to shut me up.

'I'm sorry Mr Ferris. I'm afraid your blood readings show a rise in your PSA. I...'

I didn't let him finish.

'But my PSA is 0.03. The GP said that the test showed no cause for concern.'

He spun the monitor around again.

'That's correct. Your PSA *is* now reading 0.03. Which unfortunately means it *is* now detectable. Your previous test reading was less than 0.03 and was therefore undetectable. I'm sure it is nothing to worry too much about at this stage, but we will have to monitor it closely. It could be a glitch. It could be the nerve tissue to your penis I preserved, just giving us a little positive signal. However, if we were to get another two readings where the PSA continued to rise, we would need to intervene at that stage.'

Now *he* was talking too much, and I didn't particularly like what he was saying. I had gone for the nuclear option of having my prostate removed, to cut the cancer out of my body for good. Then I could get on with my erection-less, pad-wearing new life. What was the point of allowing myself to be mutilated if it didn't mean I was cancer-free? I tried to think of some insightful questions, but my heart wasn't in it. It was in my boots instead. I did the best I could.

'What is your instinct, based on your experience, as to whether or not the PSA will rise over the next two tests, and if it does, what happens then?'

He wouldn't be drawn on hypotheticals and instead told me to let him worry about my PSA. He told me to concentrate on getting my incontinence and surgery-induced erectile dysfunction issues sorted out. I promised to double my efforts with my pelvic floor exercises. I vowed to keep trying with the Viagra. I told him I was now ready to consider all other options available to me to rouse my sleepy friend. I listened as he explained the different remedies on offer. All the solutions he described sounded hugely underwhelming to me, whether penis pump, injections, or implant. When I'd finished laughing and shaking my head, I promised half-heartedly not to dismiss any option. The thought of having to resort to any of them didn't exactly have me skipping out of his room with excitement.

Those thoughts, added to the elevated PSA reading, and ongoing incontinence issues, meant that by the time Geraldine got in from work, I was in a foul mood. She listened intently to my constant bleating without offering an opinion. When I'd finally run out of swear words and self-pity she spoke.

'Why don't we go down to the pub and have a drink?'

'Have a drink? Have a drink? Are you fucking joking me? If I have a drink I will just piss myself the whole way home. How the fuck is that going to help?'

I could see her face drop. She didn't deserve my bile. Not now. Not ever. I held my hands up.

'I'm sorry Geraldine. That was unnecessary. I'm just worried and really fed up that I don't seem to be able to get to the end of this thing. It could have been an enlarged prostate, but it was cancer instead. It could have been contained in my prostate, but there was a positive margin. The positive margin didn't have to mean my PSA would rise, but it has. I could have recovered erectile function, but I haven't. I could have been off my pads and dry, but I can't even go to the pub for a pint without pissing like a fountain.'

She leaned in and put her arms around my waist.

'And you could have had incurable pancreatic cancer, and you would be dead by now. I don't care about what we have to go through on this journey, as long as there is a journey to go on. You are still on the right side of this thing. You've had a heart attack and you have cancer. Both those things kill lots of people but you're still here and you have a chance to be here for a long time to come. That's all that matters to me and the kids. Nothing else. So what if it's not as straightforward as you had hoped? We will just have to face whatever comes.'

I wiped an offending tear from my eye and pulled her to me.

'Let's get changed and go to the pub. I'll just wear a heavier pad and black jeans. I can drink Guinness and piss to my heart's content. Who's going to know?'

CHAPTER 16

Who's going to know? Me! I'm going to know!

That's the problem. When you are dribbling urine and changing pads twice a day it's really hard to behave as if all is well in the world. *Because it isn't.* When you are leaving board meetings because your pad is feeling too heavy, then all is not well. If the last thing you do before you go out for dinner is to check that your wife has slipped a spare pad in her bag, *just in case*, it does tend to lower your mood somewhat. No matter how many times I told myself how lucky I was that I didn't have some other hideous untreatable cancer that might have killed me already, it was impossible not to feel pissed off at the latest hand I'd been dealt. I just seemed to be angry all the time. I was becoming more and more aware of how hard it must be for family and friends to be around me. Geraldine could make an innocent comment about something and I would pounce on her.

And talking of pouncing. The other sort I mean. That part of my life felt like it was over forever. Despite the mounting pile of Viagra that was now filling my kitchen cabinet, there was absolutely no sign of life down below. Just in case I give the wrong impression, I've never been in the habit of *pouncing*, but you know what I mean. One minute you're functioning perfectly normally, then after a few swishes of a surgeon's robotically guided blade you are dead as a dodo in the underpants department. Not that I wear underpants. Wait a minute? I do! I do wear underpants now. I never used to. Not for 20 years or more. Come to think of it, I have no idea why I stopped wearing them. Surely it was much more hygienic to have worn them? Anyway, I wear them now. I have to. If I don't, I have nothing to stick my pads to. There are even special sexy boxers you can buy with a built-in pad. It's quite ironic that they give you quite the bulge in your jeans while all the while hiding your dysfunctional, shrivelled, mini-me.

I was fortunate that I had other things to focus my mind on. Isla, our newly born granddaughter became the centre of my universe. She only had to be in the room for my spirits to lift, and for my mind to put the cancer, the surgery and its unpleasant side effects on the backburner. Most weekends, Conor and Kayleigh allowed us to keep her overnight on a Friday or Saturday. Her visits became the highlight of our week. Her presence took me back to happier times when I would spend hours nursing and playing with our own children. I can vividly remember when Isla's father used to sleep and slobber on my chest. The weight of him on me was a physical reminder of the enormous responsibility we all carry from the moment we become parents. I used to listen to new grandparents babbling on about the great joy a grandchild brings. If I'm honest, I would have to say I never really got it. I just couldn't understand how they could get so animated about a child who ultimately wasn't theirs. Isla coming along changed all that. I now had to bite my tongue in the office because I'd find myself wanting to tell anyone who would listen how special she was. I would often find myself, phone in hand, standing over the desk of my latest captive audience, scrolling through the photos I had taken the weekend before. My photo album had become exclusively Isla territory.

The whole grandchild thing really is something that caught me unaware and spun my world on its axis. We all have our own reasons why the mere presence of an infant in our lives turns us into the office bore. In my case, Isla came along when I was dealing with the cancer diagnosis, subsequent surgery and rising PSA. She represented hope. She symbolised the future. She lessoned my fear and tempered my feeling that the best of me and my life was already behind me. But it was more than just that. She was the first girl to come into my immediate family since my mother, Bernadette. We'd been blessed with three beautiful boys who were now young men, but I would have loved a daughter as well. Isla was a direct descendent of my mother. Just that thought was enough to make me want to hold her a little bit closer and for a little bit longer.

* * *

It was late April 2017. The upcoming publication of *The Boy on the Shed* was also something to cling on to through choppy waters. I still couldn't envisage walking into a bookshop and seeing something I'd written at my kitchen table looking back at me from the shelf. People from my background didn't write books. If they did, they certainly didn't get them published by mainstream publishers who supplied them to actual bookshops, where readers perused them before buying. They didn't harbour hopes of waking up daily to sparkling reviews from readers claiming how they just couldn't put the book down or how it was the best thing they had ever read. But that was my hope and that was my dream. Isla and the book would steer me out of the dark place I was in.

I was in a horrible place those first months after the surgery. I could feel it creeping over me like a heavy blanket. I fought against it, tried to push it off my shoulders and kick it off my feet, but I just couldn't muster the strength or the will. I would spend a day at work and it felt like a week. A job I had enjoyed so much became an uphill slog. When you are the CEO of a company you can't just slouch into the office, go through the motions, and stare at the clock until you can find a reason to leave early. Well, I say you can't, but that's exactly what I did on a daily basis for what felt like weeks on end. I tried to put a smile on my face and fake some excitement at the day's events, but I've never been much of an actor. My mood didn't go unnoticed. My friends and colleagues were all aware of my diagnosis and subsequent surgery. They were genuinely concerned for me. I stopped counting how often I was asked if everything was OK. My answer would always be the same.

I'm fine. Just a little tired.

The reality is that I wanted to scream at the person asking.

No, I'm not alright. I've only just got my head around my heart attack and having to live on lettuce for the rest of my life, now I have cancer and I can't seem to get rid of the fucker. So no, I'm not alright.

I never did offer the authentic response and the office was no doubt a happier place for that. But I wasn't happy. I would go home, have dinner and slump in the chair. I'd move only to visit the cupboard, fridge or toilet. I'd climb wearily into bed, toss and turn half the night, before getting up, trudging to work, back to the chair and back to bed. Everything seemed pointless – apart from Isla and the upcoming book publication. So, when the publishers emailed to say they had decided not to publish it in September 2017 after all, but wait until the end of February 2018, I was flattened. They asked me how I felt about the delay, was I OK with it? I replied to say *I'm fine* with it. But I wasn't. I wanted to implore them to reconsider, to beg them just to publish it on the date they promised. I wanted to tell them that my mental health depended on it. My chair, cupboard, fridge and toilet all needed a break from me. Geraldine and the kids did too. My workmates deserved better than my sour face polluting their world every day. But instead, I just said *I'm fine.* The most dishonest and useless two-word phrase ever invented. *I'm fucked. I'm empty. I'm distraught. I'm flat. I'm beaten. I'm lost* – all should be used instead of *I'm fine,* for those of us wishing to live a more authentic life. But they're also guaranteed to have friends and colleagues giving you a wide berth next time they approach you at the water cooler at work.

But friends weren't giving me a wide berth. Quite the opposite. It was me giving them a wide berth. In all circumstances, every time.

Do you fancy a pint and a catch-up?

Nah. I'm already out tonight with Geraldine.

Fancy going for dinner?

Really sorry, the in-laws are visiting.

Got a couple of tickets to the match on Saturday, do you fancy it?

I'd love to, but we are away for the weekend.

All lies and excuses. I had a million more where they came from. They just tripped off my tongue and poured out of me. I got so good at them that even I started to believe some of the imaginary plans I had made for myself. My world was shrinking and I was the cause. There are only so many times a friend will make you an offer before they just stop asking. That's exactly what happened. All the invitations stopped. No one asked anymore. So I just disappeared into my prison chair.

I'd had moments of low mood (as my doctor called it) before. That was eight or nine years previously when I'd jumped off my fledgling career as a barrister for the promise of untold riches as part of Alan Shearer's management team. It had all turned to dust before it had even begun. I'd spent a few months wallowing in self-pity at the mess I had made of my life. It had felt like I had nowhere to go. The hole I'd dug for myself was too dark and too deep. But I'd eventually fought my way back. My tools of choice (or desperation) back then were diet, exercise and sheer bloody-mindedness. I somehow had managed to find a way to carve out a new career as the boss of a health and fitness concept. So I recognised the signs. I recognised the hole that I was in danger of disappearing into again. I tried the exercise, and I tried the diet. The exercise was not as effective this time. I was a few years older than last time and my joints and muscles ached from the statin medication I was taking once more for my heart disease. I was fatter and lacked the discipline and willpower I once possessed around my diet.

By far the biggest difference between this time and last time was that I was now *sans* prostate. The effects of the surgery meant that I now wet myself while jogging, dribbled when lifting weights, and even seeped a little when doing nothing more than walking briskly. Tena For Men incontinence pads were my new best friends. I was losing all my others, so I suppose we take our friends wherever we can get them.

Viagra certainly had no interest in being my friend. Despite the hopeful mutterings of my urologist, that my spared nerves would spark back into life over time, they simply didn't materialise for me. Everything down there that had once been so familiar now felt so alien. My senses were dulled to the point that I didn't recognise the sensations I was feeling anymore. I was left with nothing more than a useless stopcock. It couldn't hold back a dribble. It was incapable of even a flicker of life no matter how many magic pills I took. I began to lose any faith that anything would ever materialise naturally from that department ever again. Such was my lack of faith that I found myself now seriously considering the options I had all but dismissed in my previous consultations.

There were the injections.

They sounded straightforward enough, if not overly pleasant. It was quite simple really. Next time the occasion arose and nothing else did, I just had to stab a needle into the base of my shaft and wait for the chemicals to lift the mood in the room. Something about the needle in my shaft just wasn't doing it for me in the early days. But after a few months of nothingness in my pants, I was now contemplating it as a viable remedy.

There were the implants.

That involved a day procedure. A reservoir would be embedded in my lower abdomen. Whatever erectile tissue I had left would be scraped away to make room for the implants. Two empty chambers would be inserted up the length of my penis. When the mood called for it, I would flick a switch discreetly hidden in my scrotum and up, up and away I'd go. Then I'd just flick the switch when I was done and revert back to my leathery alien self. If I didn't fancy the whole reservoir-and-switch-in-my-scrotum vibe, I could opt to have two flexible rods inserted instead. I'd just straighten them when I fancied it or bend them in half when I wasn't in the mood. The bendy rods hadn't taken my fancy at all when I'd first heard them mentioned. They appealed less still, the more I thought about them, even when I now knew drastic action was necessary.

There was the penis pump.

When Dr Alderton had mentioned it, I'd laughed out loud, causing him to do the same. He'd agreed with me that it sounded like something out of an *Austin Powers* movie. The thought of inserting my penis into a specially fitted vacuum pump before snapping two rings around the base of it, which stayed in place securely enough to give me an erection was hardly the stuff of great romance. Marvin wasn't contemplating that little manoeuvre when he wrote *Let's Get it On*. But this was where I now found myself. If I ever wanted to *get it on* again, then I had a clear choice between injection, implant or pump. I weighed up the pros and cons of each. There was only one winner for me.

CHAPTER 17

'Paul Ferris.'

The skinny boy shouted my name as he poked his head around the door of the waiting room. He looked 17, but I assumed he must have been at least 10 years older. He couldn't possibly be allowed to be having consultations of this nature while maybe still a virgin himself? We made some small talk as we walked past corridors of sick people slouching in chairs. I don't think hospital corridors are meant to be full of sick people; they should be in bed surely? We eventually got to his cupboard room and he asked me to sit. I can't say I was excited or filled with anticipation for the conversation to follow.

From the moment I had settled on my choice, I'd not been looking forward to this. Once I'd informed the nurse of the winner of the How to Artificially Inflate Your Reluctant Penis Competition this was the meeting I was dreading the most. Was he going to demonstrate how to use it, or worse still, was I?

'So you're here for your penis pump fitting, Mr Ferris.'

He already had the pump in his hand. My hand was sweating as he passed it to me. I wondered how many men had shared this moment with him and if they were all as apprehensive as me. Once I'd familiarised myself with the cylinder he took it back off me. I was delighted at that point but curious as to what happened next. I didn't have to wait long. He produced some lubricant and rubbed it around the tip of the cylinder. He informed me that I would need to shave my pubic hair so that the lubricant could help the cylinder form a tight seal around the base of my penis. He emphasised how important it was that I didn't trap my testicles in the vacuum. *I mean, who wants to*

do that? I knew a man once who'd had to go to the hospital cos he'd…
anyway, never mind. My instructor skilfully slipped what can only
accurately be described as a cock ring around the lubricated pump.
He then slipped another one over it for good measure. He held it up
to my face and told me I had to slide it over my penis. One startled
look from me later, he reassured me he didn't mean there and then.
He meant when I got home. I relaxed. *He probably didn't even mean
immediately after I got home. I could probably have my dinner first.
Maybe watch* Line of Duty, *before informing Geraldine with a wink
that I was off to the bathroom. Maybe ask her to give me 10 minutes
or so.*

He was a really nice lad. He was very professional and acutely
aware of the embarrassment and anxiety coming from my side of his
office. He took time to explain what I could expect and problems
I may have. He was so committed to his product that I practically
skipped out of his office in eager anticipation of my first erection
since losing my prostate. He'd been so convincing in his belief that all
my problems in the penis department were solved that I couldn't wait
to share my new toy with Geraldine. *Line of Duty* would have to wait.
I'd probably still have my dinner first though.

As it happens, I had several dinners. I'd wanted to try it but part
of me was frightened that it wouldn't work, or worse still, that it
would, but my bits would look like a choked chicken and Geraldine
would reject me. How bloody stupid is that? To have the solution to a
problem right there in your lap and then to let fear get in the way of
your potential path to a better place? No matter how silly you know
you are being, it still doesn't stop the procrastination and sabotage.
Certainly, in my case, that is an all too familiar truth. Several times in
my life I have found myself close to the finishing line of a project, all
the hard work done, only to blow the whole thing. I mean how hard
can it be to pump up your own penis?

Three weeks after bringing it home I finally plucked up the courage
to try. I waited till everyone was out of the house and made my way
upstairs and got the pump out of the bathroom cupboard in which I'd
hidden it. Using it was quite the challenge. After shaving, lubricating

and stretching the cock rings over the cylinder, I was ready to go. I slipped my sorry self into the tube, made sure the lubricated rubber was attached to my newly shaved skin, and began to pump the lever. It sealed immediately and two or three pumps later I could see signs of life in the tube. My joy was abruptly halted when I felt a sharp searing pain in my left testicle. I was frozen in agony for what felt like minutes, but was probably seconds, before my fingers found their way to the little red button that released the vacuum pressure and with it, my poor trapped testicle, which had found its way into the vacuum before I had started the procedure. Undaunted, and with great dexterity – pump and lever in one hand, stray testicle in the other – I began again. It really was miraculous. Every pump was a joy to behold until my erect penis pushed itself against the glass cylinder. That was my signal to stop pumping, according to my skinny friend. I stood in silent awe and studied my gloriously hard penis. Not a sentence I'd ever envisaged speaking in my life, never mind writing. And one, when taken out of context, has the enormous potential to make me look like a bit of a bell-end. I trust you will forgive me the indulgence just this once.

My wondrous joy was dramatically curtailed the moment the first ring slipped off the vacuum tube and snapped tightly around the base of my now slightly deflated offering. The pain was immense and not helped by the fact that my foreskin was pulled sharply downwards by the vice-like grip of the ring. I wiped my watering eyes and dutifully followed the procedure I'd been shown. I tucked the ring inside the tube and ensured it was sealed against my shaven skin. Undeterred, but a little warily, I pumped gently again. My strangled semi-erect penis responded. Only this time it was throbbing as it got harder – and not in a good way. For a brief moment I thought about aborting the whole thing and sending the pump and rings straight back to where they came from. Yet it had been so long since I'd seen any signs of life down there that the thought of the potential pleasure at the end of the process overrode any pain I was feeling. I remembered my skinny friend telling me something about lots of men pumping up their bits too much in the desire to have a bigger erection. He'd warned me not to fall into that trap. As I'd looked down at my swollen and aching erection, I'd clearly fallen into the same ego-driven trap. I fiddled for the little button and released the pressure. It wasn't quite bliss. I still had a ring clamped vice-like at the bottom of my shaft. But it was at least tolerable pain again. I pumped gently once more until I was satisfied with the level of throbbing and slipped the hard plastic ring off the vacuum.

Jesus Christ the Night!

I hopped around the bathroom for a few seconds, stood on the discarded pump and stubbed my toe on the toilet. All the while my twice-strangled penis was half-standing to attention and turning from red to purple. I tried to ride it out, to wait for the pain to subside, but it just didn't. If anything, it got worse. I hobbled over to the bed, lay down on my back and tried to get the rings off as fast as I could. I pulled them sideways and longways until they made their way up to the tip of my penis. They both flew off in different directions as they finally gave up their torturing of my poor bits. I lay for a second in blessed relief that they were gone.

I picked up the box that housed the vacuum pump. I looked at the smiling, handsome grey-haired couple holding hands in the leafy glade. The photo cut off at the top of the man's waistband. I was pretty sure by his relaxed smile and contented gaze that he wasn't wearing his cock rings when the photographer snapped that particular moment. In fact, I was certain no one would ever smile again if they'd just had their bits trapped by those vicious little bastards.

I slipped the vacuum, rings and lubricant into the neat little zip up bag and stuffed the bag in the cupboard. I walked to the bed and thought about climbing in. I looked at the clock. 5.15 p.m. was a bit early, even for me, these days. It would have taken a bit of explaining to Geraldine that everything was fine in my world if she'd come home from work to find me and my recently strangled penis tucked up for the night.

But that was just it. Everything wasn't fine in my world. How could it be? I'd just spent the past 20 minutes trying and failing to pump myself an erection. Even if I'd been successful in my endeavours then the end result from what I'd just seen wasn't even a stuffable one. And just supposing it was actually stuffable, the orgasm at the end of it would be a dry one anyway. No prostate – no semen. *A dry orgasm.* Now wasn't that something to look forward to.

I felt a mixture of sorrow, frustration and disappointment that my latest efforts with the pump hadn't enabled me to achieve an erection. Then I was annoyed with myself for letting that failure affect my mood so much. I reminded myself that every day there were lots of men diagnosed with late-stage prostate cancer who would have swapped places with me right there and then. Those men, who were only diagnosed after the disease had spread to other parts of their bodies, could probably still get their erections but they were living with a death sentence. I was just living with having to change some aspects of my life. What's a permanently flaccid penis and a few dribbles of piss into a pad compared to facing death and extinction? I snapped myself out of it and made my way downstairs.

I bumped into Geraldine at the bottom on her way up.

'What are you doing home so early?'

I was grateful she hadn't arrived 10 minutes earlier.

'I'm not early. I always get home at this time. What have you been up to?'

'Me. Nothing. Why. Who are you? The Gestapo or something?'

She was startled by my tone. I was startled by my tone.

'Alright. Jesus. I was only asking how your day went. No need to bite my head off.'

And she was. She was just a wife asking a husband a routine question after we'd both arrived home after a long day at work. The trouble was, I was just a husband who'd only moments before packed away my vacuum pump and cock rings. A husband whose poor strangled penis was still stinging from the experience.

I should have just answered her question. I should have just told her what I had been up to. We had no secrets from each other, and she had been my wife for 29 years. Why should I be embarrassed? I was just being ridiculously stupid. I should just have told her about my efforts. After all, it was for her benefit, too – I'm sure she couldn't wait to be confronted with one of my new cock-ring-supported-vacuum-pumped-stuffable erections. Why shouldn't I tell her of my progress in that department? It's not as if she had come home and found me in bed with someone, or maybe watching porn with my semen-filled-cock-ring-free cock in my hand. I was merely following medical advice. Of course I should tell her. I would bloody tell her. Right here. Right now.

'Sorry Geraldine, I was just… I was just… I was just…'

'Jesus Paul. Spit it out will you? You're worrying me now. Is everything alright?'

'Yes. Yes. I was just. Well. I was…'

'Your face is beetroot red. Are you OK?'

'OK? Me? Yes. I'm great. If you would just let me get a word in. I was just seeing if our passports are in date. I was thinking we should book a holiday. We've had a tough year and all that and I thought it would be nice if we…'

She hugged me.

'Oh, that's fantastic. I wanted to suggest it but wasn't sure you would be up for it. Are they in date?'

'Are what in date?'

'Jesus, Paul. The passports. Are they in date?'

'Oh those. Yeah, they are in date.'

'That's great. I thought mine was due a renewal?'

'Err… I will check again. I just had a quick glance at them. But we have plenty of time if it's not.'

She turned and headed towards the kitchen. I followed, annoyed with myself for being embarrassed about something I shouldn't need to be embarrassed about. I resolved to tell her about the pump thing after dinner. We sat down with a glass of wine two hours later. The perfect time to tell her? *Maybe not.* Three hours later we'd booked a holiday to Florence, Venice and Rome. She was none the wiser for my efforts in the pump department.

We climbed into bed. I kissed her goodnight and turned my back to her.

'How did you get on with the vacuum pump today?'

'What?'

How the hell could she know about that?

'Today, when you were checking the passports, how did you get on?'

'Not great. How did you know I was doing that?'

She turned around and held her hand up to my face.

'I found one of these ring things on my dressing table when I came up to get changed after dinner. Why didn't you just tell me? There is nothing to be embarrassed about.'

I took it from her.

'Wait a minute. That means you knew before I went ahead and booked the holiday? I only did that cos I'd lied about the passports.'

She smiled in the darkness and kissed me.

'I'm many things, but I'm not stupid. And now we are going to Italy. That's a pretty good day's work on my part I'd say.'

I leaned in and kissed her. Then I made love to my wife for the first time since having my prostate removed. Who needs injections, implants, pumps, cock rings – or erections for that matter? I held her in my arms until she fell asleep on my chest. Then I had my best night's sleep since my surgery.

CHAPTER 18

The holiday to Italy was something to look forward to. Something else for me to focus on, other than my health issues. For as long as I can remember I've always been prone to overthinking things. Added to that, I have a tendency to develop low moods which I can trace back to my mother's death in 1987. It's fair to say that in the early summer of 2017, some five months after my prostatectomy, I was probably as low as I have ever been. The surgery hadn't worked and my PSA was rising. My incontinence pads were still getting a daily soaking, and my surgically induced erectile dysfunction troubled me more than I cared to admit – even to Geraldine. It's a very unsettling thing when something that you'd taken for granted all your life is suddenly ripped away from you. But it was more than that. Much more – the loss of this essential part of me was soul-crushing.

I tried again to throw myself into my work in the hope that the distraction and the normality would snap me out of the blackness. I tried more exercise, too. Neither worked. The more I tried to re-engage with work the more exhausted I was when I got home. On several occasions on my way home from work I had to pull the car over to the side of the road. The tiredness that enveloped me was so all-consuming that I knew if I hadn't, I was a danger to myself and other drivers. When I did get home, I'd quickly make dinner. Then I'd slump into the chair for the remainder of the night. My night would end with Geraldine getting fed up with me sleeping through our favourite programmes and she'd usher me off to bed.

There was nothing that could lift my mood. Well, not quite nothing. One thing could lift my spirits in an instant. Not a thing exactly. More a tiny bundle of miracle that was guaranteed to get me off my chair and smile just in anticipation of seeing her. I began to look forward to her visits so much that I started to worry I was becoming a bit obsessed with this little girl, who'd come into my life just when I needed her the most. She was five months old now and recognised the important people in her life. She'd signal that recognition with beaming gums and limbs flailing. When I looked into her eyes and she smiled into mine, the connection was cloud-busting. I am not a believer in a higher power, but if I were, I would swear Isla was sent as a beacon of hope just when I needed it most.

Music, too, could still lift me. Not all the time, but when I was in the mood, the right song could transport me back to my youth. A place where ill health and fear of dying were matters for the old people to worry about. Occasionally, on a Friday night, we could be found drinking wine and reminiscing into the night about the significant events of our courtship and our early years together. All those old familiar songs provided the backdrop to those nights. They were capable of instantly transporting me to a happier time and place. The wine helped, too. I remember once reading about a scientific study that highlighted the age at which we stop listening to new music and instead listen exclusively to the songs of our past. Whatever age it was, I had long passed through it. Van Morrison, Irish folk, rock and blues, and a bit of soul, would be the dominant theme of those drunken nights.

But the respite that Isla and the music provided weren't enough to entirely dig me out of the hole I was in. On my last visit to the GP he had asked how I was getting on. I'd mentioned that my mood was low and that this was my main concern. I'd expected my revelation might lead to some further intervention, such as a recommendation of therapy maybe. None was forthcoming. Instead, we moved on to something else entirely and I left the consultation no further forward in trying to find a solution for how I was feeling. For now, it would have to be Isla, music and the upcoming holiday to Italy that would provide temporary respite and relief from the darkness that threatened to consume me.

Even the anticipation of the holiday was tempered by the fact that I was to have my latest blood test done soon after returning. The one that would confirm whether or not I had indeed suffered a 'biochemical failure'. If my surgery hadn't worked, I would require hormone therapy and radiotherapy to try and halt the march of this stubborn invader. I had watched from afar as my brother-in-law Kieran had undergone both treatments. It hadn't looked very pleasant from my vantage point. More importantly though, it did seem to be doing the trick for him. Surgery hadn't been an option for him because by the time of his diagnosis, the cancer had spread beyond his prostate.

I called him. I listened on the phone as he reeled off the side effects of the radiotherapy – fatigue, chronic diarrhoea, urinary incontinence and erectile problems. I was already living with two of those unwelcome visitors, so wasn't too bothered about adding the others. He told me his hormone therapy had given him a very nice pair of breasts and had cost him any libido he'd previously possessed. The potential growth of my breasts didn't bother me too much but the thought of losing my libido certainly did. It was bad enough not being able to generate an erection of any kind without strangling my penis to death. But at least I still possessed the urge to try. I couldn't, and didn't, want to imagine a life where that urge was non-existent. It seemed absurdly harsh to me. I was 52, not 22, but I still felt young – as strange as that sounds from someone who'd suffered a heart attack at 48 and had prostate cancer by 51. I still felt relatively fit, apart from the obvious changes down below.

As time passed after my surgery the physical challenges were no longer my only concern. They were matched, and sometimes surpassed by my delicate mental state. I needed something to stop my descent. I just didn't know what that was until one evening when I was working on my laptop, slouched in my chair. I don't even know how I ended up staring at a newly opened Word document, but there it was, right in front of me, offering me an escape from the pit of despair I'd found myself in.

'Are you coming to bed?'

When I finally looked up from the keyboard I'd been furiously tapping at, Geraldine was standing over me with a glass of water and mobile phone in hand.

'What. It's not that late is it? What time is it?'

'It's midnight. You haven't lifted your head from that screen for the last three hours. What are you doing anyway?'

Midnight? I stared at the flickering screen in front of me. I scrolled to the top of the typo-riddled mess I had been working on. The top of the page read, *A Week in September.* Below that, there were 3,000 words that represented the beginning of a new book I had begun subconsciously more than three hours before. I felt a surge of adrenalin. My head was buzzing with possibilities. I didn't like the title, but it would do for now. It wasn't about the title. It wasn't even about the words on the page. It was about the three hours that had just evaporated without me once thinking about cancer, radiotherapy, hormone treatment or all the other nonsense that had been slowly robbing me of my mental wellbeing. I had found my escape route.

I turned the screen so Geraldine could see my latest handiwork. She slipped onto the chair next to me and began reading all about Jeff Smith and Chris Scott, two individuals that hadn't existed three hours ago but who were now about to tear each other's imaginary worlds apart. All in the name of my sanity. And that is exactly what they did, any time I had some spare time. Instead of ruminating on where life had taken me, I simply took myself out of my troubled head and into an entirely new world. When I wasn't writing, I was thinking about writing, and when I was thinking about writing, I wasn't thinking about cancer.

It is hard to describe the satisfaction I got, and still get, from putting random words together on a page. When I'm writing, everything feels right in my world. I have no expectations that anyone will ever read what I write. It's just the process I like. When I'm writing I find it really hard to be anything other than exhilarated, happy and alive. How can something as simple as putting words on a page bring so much joy? I don't know and I don't care. I'm just relieved and thankful that it does.

A Week in September became *An Ugly Game,* and Jeff and Chris grew to be as much a part of my daily life as sleeping, washing and eating. They gave me rest from the restlessness of worrying about the uncertain future I was facing. They gave Geraldine peace from my misery. They gave my kids back their father. I was no longer the angst-ridden mess who slumped defeated on the chair the moment he arrived home from work. We took Owen and Ciaran to Italy with us – Pisa to Florence to Venice to Rome to Cinque Terre. All by train, and all journeys passed in a blur of writing and more writing. While the others slept, I wrote, stopping only when the breath-taking Italian countryside we were speeding through forced me to pause for a moment and let its impossible beauty wash over me. Venice and Florence were like nothing I'd ever experienced before. The history, the architecture, the sounds, the smells. I loved all of it. Drinking wine and people-watching in St Mark's Square in the evening. Inhaling the soft orchestral music that made its way from all corners of the piazza and seeped into my bones. Seeing the smiles on the faces of Geraldine and my boys as we stared intoxicated by the setting sun over the Ponte Vecchio. We stayed for three weeks. I could have stayed forever.

By the time we got back, I had written 50,000 words and the darkness of the previous months had disappeared into my keyboard. I felt ready to take on the world again and went back to work with a spring in my step. I had a renewed determination to repay Graham Wylie for his unwavering belief in me, and his quiet support. Not just through the cancer diagnosis and treatment, but also for his reassurance after my heart attack in 2013. He'd been the first person to visit me when I returned from hospital on both occasions. Both times his message had been the same:

'It's your company. Take as long as you need to recover. It will all be here for you when you feel well enough to come back.'

He'd delivered his messages with no fanfare, no grand gestures. He was just a caring man doing a decent thing for another human being who was vulnerable and in need of help. I was desperate to repay that faith. And since I now had the book to focus my fragile mind on in the evenings, I could throw myself back into my work during the day. Life was good again. So good, I nearly forgot to get my blood test done in time for my follow-up appointment with the urologist. I managed to beg the receptionist at the GP to squeeze me in at very short notice, otherwise my appointment with the consultant two days later would have been completely pointless. Thankfully, she heeded my desperate pleading. I got my bloods done in time, and saw Dr Alderton as planned. He shook my hand and offered me a seat. Then he delivered some news I didn't want to hear.

'Your PSA has doubled since your last visit. That is three rising results since your surgery. That indicates a biochemical failure from your surgery. I have booked you an appointment with the oncologist for as soon as possible. You will start radiotherapy shortly after. Meanwhile, I have written you a prescription for hormone treatment that I want you to start today.'

He explained further.

'Both treatments do produce side effects. You may get one or all of them. The hormone treatment will mean you will grow some breast tissue and you will have no libido. The radiotherapy will destroy the nerves we spared to your penis and will severely restrict your ability to have a natural erection in the future. The treatment can also make your incontinence worse and can lead to short- or long-term bowel issues.'

I wanted to scream out with frustration and anger. *The mutilating surgery hadn't been enough after all. The sepsis and the anaemia had been for nothing. The erectile dysfunction and the incontinence that had so detrimentally affected my quality of life were not going to improve. If anything, they were going to get worse. If the radiotherapy and hormone treatment didn't work. What next?*

I didn't scream out in the end. Instead, I just resigned myself to my fate. I left his room with a weak smile and a handshake. I walked to the car park on unsteady legs. I made it to the car before the first tears escaped. I cried like a child for 10 minutes before wiping my nose. I called Geraldine.

'Well, how did it go?'

I tried to speak but couldn't. She spoke for me.

'I'm leaving work now; I will see you at home. Whatever it is, we will deal with it. I love you.'

Someone knocked on the car window. I lowered it.

'Are you staying or going mate? I've been blocking half the car park waiting for you to leave.'

He was agitated, impatient and rude. His tone felt unnecessarily abrupt to me. In other circumstances and on another day, I'd have let him know that. Not today. Instead, I raised my wet hands and apologised. I left him and his anger in the car park. I made my way to Geraldine.

CHAPTER 19

All of my urology appointments had been in the main hospital. My oncology appointment letter informed me my new journey was to begin in different territory. As I made my way along the sterile corridors, I passed busy nurses, important looking doctors, patients in wheelchairs, or pushing their trolleys with saline hanging from it. I left the older part of the hospital behind me and found myself standing at the pristine counter of the new wing. The sign behind the desk told me I was in the right place. *The Northern Centre For Cancer Care.*

I had been here when I was having my bone scans just before Christmas the year before. I hoped I would never be back and my surgery was meant to ensure that was the case. This wing of the hospital had been built in 2009 and proudly boasted of its award-winning record in helping patients beat cancer and leukaemia. As I stood waiting for the busy woman in glasses to lift her head and acknowledge me, I wished this place was helping someone else other than me to beat cancer. Standing in a dedicated cancer care unit felt more sinister than visiting the urologist's office. There, I was just another of his patients, some had urinary tract infections, some had enlarged prostates, others had kidney stones. In this place, I was a cancer sufferer, just like everyone else hovering miserably around the reception area, but I didn't want to be that. Whoever wants to be that? When I was running around the playground, or a football pitch, without a care in the world, days like these seemed so far away that I couldn't have ever envisaged how they might feel. But now those days were here. And they felt worse than anything my childhood imagination was capable of conjuring. They felt dark, empty, soulless and scary.

'Can I help you?'

The glasses behind reception were pointing in my direction.

I mumbled something back to her. Mumbling has become a new bad habit of mine. If I find myself at a counter, any counter – it could be the doctors, butchers, chip shop or travel agents – as soon as the person on the other side asks, 'can I help you?' it's like my brain instantly stops communicating with my mouth. Instead of a confident 'could I please have', or 'could you direct me to', I transform myself into a jabbering, whispering blushing mess. I don't know why it happens, but it always does. Maybe it's an adult manifestation of my crushing shyness as a boy? I've no idea why I react in that way. I get annoyed with myself for doing it. The net effect is always an uncomfortable standoff while the poor person on the other side of my performance tries again to get the information needed to answer my query.

'You're in the right building but at the wrong desk. You need oncology outpatients. It's back along the corridor behind you, then turn right at the end.'

Her glasses were back focussing on the screen in front of her. Glad to be rid of me no doubt. I looked once more at my appointment letter. The first line in bold read, *Oncology Outpatients*. I followed the signs dotted on the ceiling above me as I walked along. They all pointed me quite clearly towards the *Oncology Department*. How is it possible to go through this life and not be able to correctly follow the simple instructions on an appointment letter? I arrived at the reception and mumbled to a new victim behind the counter before taking my seat in the overcrowded waiting room. A very helpful neon sign on the wall informed me that all of the doctors were on time. All apart from mine. Mine was operating on a 40-minute delay. I looked around for something to read. After 10 minutes of reading leaflets on *Cancer and Family, Cancer and Exercise, Cancer and Nutrition, Cancer and Benefits, Cancer and Sex, Cancer and Wig Fitting*, I'd had more than enough of *Cancer and Everything*. I looked around the room and saw a familiar face. It was a friend of a friend. I'd been in his company a few times over the years. He was an Irishman, who'd always had a ready smile and a handshake when our paths crossed. I thought about going over to speak with him, to ask him how life was treating him, but I knew by the look on his face how that conversation would go.

'What you doing here?'

'Cancer.'

'Me too.'

'Great. How's the family?'

It wasn't a chat that I fancied having. I picked up another cancer leaflet and hid behind that until my name was called.

Dr Frew called my name as he appeared at the edge of the waiting area. He was a familiar, friendly face from when I'd been weighing up my options after the initial shock of my diagnosis. I'd made the decision to opt for surgery in the hope that I'd never have to see him, or any other oncologist, ever again. That 'foolproof' course of action hadn't worked out so well. We made small talk as we entered his office and I positioned myself at the side of his desk. I felt at ease with him. He had a ready smile, a keen interest in sport, and seemed genuinely fascinated by my efforts in writing *The Boy on the Shed* and its upcoming publication. He had an air of quiet confidence about him that was a perfect antidote to the fear and uncertainty that I carried into his room.

He browsed my notes, looked at the screen and studied my notes again. I felt sick that I had to be here with him. My plan had been to have surgery, cure cancer and move on. But here I was, still with cancer, and waiting for the oncologist to tell me what my chances were of ever getting rid of it. I sat patiently staring into space. He hummed and murmured to himself and finally settled on a way forward to give me a chance of doing just that. When he was satisfied, he lifted his head and rocked back on his chair. I felt my pulse quicken as he delivered his verdict on my future prospects.

'You are an interesting one.'

I took that to be a positive start.

'I see lots of men here in your situation who have had a biochemical failure.'

I wasn't too keen on the 'failure' part.

'I usually recommend hormone treatment and a course of salvage radiotherapy. In truth, I do so with a heavy heart in lots of cases. It's a bit like shutting the stable door after the horse has bolted. The cancer is no longer contained in the capsule. But in your case...'

He was leaning forward now and rubbing his chin. He was warming to his task.

'In your case it's different. You are an intriguing prospect.'

It's always good to be intriguing.

'You had a less than a one-millimetre positive margin on your biopsy, with a Gleason 3 at the margin. The chances of cure after a biochemical failure are usually around 50/50, but I think in your case it's better than that.'

A good chance he could get it!

When he had finished speaking my fear had become something else. Hope, belief – excitement even. I might still be one of the lucky ones after all.

I could have reached over the desk and kissed him for giving me hope. But hope was all he had given me. Hope was fantastic and better than lots of people in my situation get. But I wanted more. I wanted certainty. I wanted the certainty I'd had before the surgery. Granted it had proved to be nothing more than a mirage, but that feeling of security, knowing that curing my cancer was an option, was a feeling I was desperate to have again. I thought it had gone when the surgery had failed. But sitting in the oncologist's office the possibility of a cure was back on the table. I was excited by that. But as quickly as the hope and excitement had risen the clawing doubts took hold. They clawed and climbed their way to the surface. Nagging questions filled my head. I needed to ask them. They were no doubt the result of too many hours browsing the internet. Too much time spent reading the 'Sword

of Damocles' ramblings of Brad in Massachusetts and his army of
doom-mongers. According to them, once the 'genie was out of the
bottle' and the cancer was outside my prostate, then it was only
a matter of waiting for the 'hammer to fall'. My PSA would rise
again as the cancer moved around my body. So many miserable
metaphors – all pointing me towards my impending doom. I
shared my fears with Dr Frew.

'That all sounds great but what happens if I have the treatment and
the PSA rises again and we don't get it? Does that mean I will never
get rid of it?'

He smiled knowingly at the question he must have been asked a
thousand times by worried faces staring into his. He delivered his
response with total confidence.

'Then we try something else.'

He raised his hands.

'I have more tricks up my sleeve. If we don't get the result we want
from this treatment, then we try something else. If that doesn't work,
then we try something else again. This is a long journey you are on
regardless of what happens after this course of treatment. You are not
going anywhere anytime soon.'

His last sentence eased my mind in an instant. It was delivered
with such calm assurance that it was also enough for me to know
that I had found the right man to guide me through this unfamiliar
terrain.

With my doubts firmly assuaged we then discussed the best time
to commence my 33 sessions of radiotherapy and the possible side
effects I could expect. I told him the upcoming publication date for
The Boy on the Shed was 22 February 2018. He said I could wait until
publication and have the radiotherapy after that date. He told me my
hormone treatment was already dampening any cancerous activity
and would continue to do so until then. I asked him if I could get
it out of the way before publication. I hated the idea of having what
promised to be one of the greatest moments of my life tarnished.
The fact that I would have the upcoming treatment looming on
the horizon would undoubtedly spoil what enjoyment I might get

from having a book published. He was incredibly helpful and as determined as me that I was going to have my moment in the sun, without my cancer getting in the way of everything. We settled on radiotherapy treatment every day over the Christmas and the New Year period with two days off – one for Christmas Day 2017 and one for New Year's Day 2018. It wasn't a prospect that thrilled me. Should I experience some of the side effects he outlined – cramps, diarrhoea, urinary incontinence, pain on micturition (peeing) and tiredness – it would certainly make for an interesting holiday season. I didn't really care about that. I'd spent Christmas 2016 having bone scans in a deserted outpatient clinic. A few more visits this Christmas would be worth it so that I could really enjoy the upcoming book release.

I met the prostate specialist nurse on my way out of the oncology department.

'How are you getting on Paul?'

She knew my name? I was impressed by that. Given the number of patients she must be looking after I thought it was impressive to remember the name of someone she had met on only one or two occasions. I fully intended to tell her I was doing well, before rushing off to fight with some impatient bastard in the car park, but before I knew it, I was sitting in her office talking about things I hadn't even discussed with Geraldine. After half an hour of discussing sex – the lack of it, the lack of ability to perform it, the lack of desire to even try it – all my barriers were down. Anything was up for discussion, however uncomfortable I felt about it.

'Have you considered a penile implant Paul?'

What? Not really. No.

I had dismissed it previously. That was before I'd opted for strangling my penis with cock rings and pumps.

I shuffled in my chair and stared at her knees.

'I haven't really considered that option, no.'

I could feel her gaze on the top of my head.

'I really think you should think about it. I find myself recommending this route to lots of men in your situation – younger men post-prostatectomy – who have not recovered erectile function.'

137

Erectile function. Erectile recovery. Erectile dysfunction. No matter how many times I heard those terms they never sounded any better. In fact, I hated them. I hated that I hadn't considered them enough before my surgery. I'd been so keen to get the cancer cut out that I hadn't given enough thought to how the subsequent side effects would alter my physical state. I had also totally underestimated the profound impact on my mental state. Since the first moment I'd realised that my bits were no longer playing the game, I'd felt an uneasiness about the future that I just couldn't shake. My inability to have an erection was something that occupied my thoughts at some point every single day. I wasn't spending all day every day thinking about it, but I was spending some time every day dwelling on it. Now I was having a very in-depth conversation with a nurse who was telling me how to rectify it. She provided me with more information than I had previously had on both types of implant.

'There are two main options. One is to have two pliable rods inserted in the shaft of your penis. When you wish to have an erection you straighten the rods and when you don't you bend them down. But they are permanently there.'

I hadn't warmed to that option when it had been mentioned to me before. It hadn't sounded great then. It sounded no less horrific when she discussed it here.

'I don't think I fancy that one to be honest. Could you explain the other option in a bit more detail?'

She spent the next 10 minutes describing the reservoir that would be inserted in my abdomen, the on-off switch positioned in my scrotal sac, and the cylinders up the shaft of my penis. She discussed infections, failures, corrective surgery and the possible need for replacement after 10 years. By the time she'd finished I was pretty sure that whatever the future held for my reluctant penis, it didn't involve rods, cylinders, switches or reservoirs. I would go home and discuss the alternatives with Geraldine. Maybe she would have a different view?

CHAPTER 20

Geraldine didn't show much enthusiasm for the bend-it-straighten-it-at-will willy. She was all too aware of my tendency to be forgetful. She had a genuine concern, that one day I might forget to bend it at the appropriate time and get arrested for offending public decency. I assured her, that even for me, that was unlikely to happen. I couldn't guarantee it though! She was, however, slightly more enthusiastic about the reservoir in the abdomen, flick the switch, cylinders up the shaft one. She didn't quite champion it enough for me to go rushing back to the nurse and ask her to book me in. Because Geraldine didn't push matters, and I really didn't fancy the idea of another surgery after my sepsis and anaemia as a result of my last one, I decided to leave things as they were and just do nothing. It wasn't dismissed entirely, but it was well and truly parked for the moment. I suppose I hoped that everyday life would take over and I could forget all about my downstairs problems.

Life did take over, but not the everyday sort. Christmas 2017 was fast approaching and just like Christmas the year before, mine would be spent visiting the Northern Centre for Cancer Care. Last year, it had been to have the bone scan to establish whether or not my cancer had already escaped my prostate, which would have made the idea of surgery redundant. This year, my visit was so that I could undergo a CT scan. The aim was to accurately pinpoint my prostate bed now that there was no prostate resting in it. This was to ensure my upcoming daily radiotherapy sessions would hit the right spot. It was a Friday in mid-December when I arrived for the last appointment of the day. They were running very late. Two hours later I was the only person left in the barely lit basement. The overworked and seriously delayed radiographer had already been out twice to apologise before her colleague finally came out and sat down beside me.

He had a peculiar looking pouch in his hand, a small cube with a long, thin neck stretching from it. I'd seen something like it before. He saw me staring at it and lifted it up, so it was at eye level for both of us. Then he outlined what I could expect from my radiotherapy experience.

'We'll be taking you into the scanner shortly where you will just need to lie still. My colleague will ink three small tattoos on you. That's to make sure any radiographer who's treating you can accurately place you in the same position each time you visit for your upcoming treatments. Your bladder should be full for each visit. So you will drink a cup of water 30 minutes before each session.'

He looked again at the long-necked capsule he was holding. I knew its destination before he told me.

'Your bowels will also need to be empty on every visit I'm afraid. That's where my friend here comes into play. Have you ever had an enema in the past?'

'Yes. I had one before my surgery. Before that I had one about 10 years ago.'

The one I'd had before my prostatectomy wasn't too bad as far as enemas go. But the one I'd had 10 years before still gave me nightmares. It was the mother of all enemas. I'd been booked in for a colonoscopy. The night before the procedure I'd been advised to drink some liquid that would clear my bowels in preparation. Twenty minutes after taking it my stomach convulsed in excruciating spasms and I barely made it to the bathroom before the violent explosions torpedoed our toilet for the next 15 minutes. Each evacuation was preceded by the most brutally painful cramps. I had hoped never to have another one, although the one before the surgery hadn't been as bad as the first. I told him about both enema experiences. He smiled.

'Don't worry. This one will be more like your most recent one. In fact, it may be a little gentler than that one even.'

I was reassured by his words.

'You just screw the top off, slide it in, and squeeze the contents out. Then wait for it to get to work.'

That seemed straightforward enough. Nothing to worry about.

He wasn't finished.

'You will then need to take one before each of your radiotherapy sessions. Not all 33. Just the first 22.'

Twenty-two enemas? Jesus Christ!

With that cheery news, he left me with my thoughts and a box of 23 enemas. I slipped into the nearest bathroom. It was a mildly unpleasant experience squirting the contents of the first capsule up my bum. I hovered around outside the toilet as I was frightened to move too far away, just in case. At the first sign of a cramp, I was trousers down, hovering over the bowl, filled with dread of what was to come. But he was right, it wasn't nearly as bad as my first experience and more akin to my second one. Not too bad on the whole, though I would hardly recommend it. The thought of another 22 didn't fill me with great joy either.

Bowels successfully evacuated, I was ushered into the room that housed the CT scanner. Two middle-aged radiographers greeted me. My friend, with the stash of enemas, had gone home. The two weary women looked like they would rather be anywhere else but there at 8 p.m. on a Friday night.

'I hope I'm not keeping you back from your night out?'

The older one answered.

'I'm at that age where I no longer have them, but I'm sure she has something planned.'

She nodded towards her colleague, who didn't break stride.

'I have something planned, but it's not until later, so I have plenty of time.'

The way she rushed around, moving me from one position to another, I suspected she had less time than she had said. It was a boring and painless affair and I eventually found myself back outside in the darkness of winter, making my way to the car in the freezing cold. I turned the engine on and ramped up the heating. John Lennon sprung to life on the radio singing about war being over. This year, like the one before it, I just wasn't in the mood for him. I was all out of Christmas spirit again. I turned him off on the first chorus and drove home with the noise of the windscreen wipers working hard on the sleet and rain bouncing off my window. Thirty-three sessions of radiotherapy and 22 enemas to look forward to, running through Christmas and finishing at the end of January. Not a prospect to fill anyone with festive joy. But there was always my book launch to look forward to. The date for publication in late February was within touching distance. Dr Frew said I might still be experiencing some side effects from the treatment by the time of publication but it would be nothing that I couldn't manage. After all, what's a bit of urinary incontinence, diarrhoea and fatigue when you have a book launch to look forward to?

I remember very little about Christmas 2017, which is weird. I mean, I was definitely there, present and enjoying the season with the rest of my family. Yet I can remember barely a bit of it. I don't know what presents I bought my children; I can't recall what nights out we had. I don't recall how much eating and drinking I did. I can't recollect what we did on Christmas Eve. I can't remember Christmas Day, whether or not I fell asleep after dinner, or if we played games or watched a movie. I do remember three things though. My nipples hurt. My breasts grew bigger. And I remember my radiotherapy appointments.

I wasn't exactly body beautiful before the hormone treatment, but my body was changing rapidly – and not for the better. It seemed like overnight I had become the not-so-proud owner of two good handfuls of breast tissue. Then there were my nipples. Back at school, we'd gone through a phase of nipping each other's nipples. Not just nipping them but nipping and twisting. Nipping and twisting nipples while shouting 'Jack the Diddy Nipper,' at the poor victim rubbing his recently assaulted nipples. After being that victim on one too many occasions, mine had developed large lumps underneath them. When I was 13, they became so swollen, that I had to pay an embarrassing visit to the doctor. Taking my shirt off in front of him and my mother was one of the most cringe-worthy moments of my adolescence. Now the pain, tenderness and embarrassment of those distant days was with me once more. My nipples were getting bigger. The bigger they got, the more painful they became. Jack the Diddy Nipper had come for me once again.

Initially, I was extremely self-conscious of my enlarged nipples and blossoming bosom. I would hide them from Geraldine. But then as the weeks passed, I began to let them hang out with the rest of the 'new' me. When I occasionally stopped and looked in the mirror, I no longer recognised the distorted image looking back at me. I'd gained weight. I'd acquired five scars that looked like stab wounds and a mangled belly button courtesy of my surgery and now I was in possession of two throbbing nipples perched on two ever-growing breasts. After weeks of tormenting myself in the mirror I got to the point where I really couldn't take anymore demoralization and self-loathing. So I simply stopped looking.

The radiotherapy appointments started in late December. Bleak days in every way for me. It's hard to get into the spirit of Christmas when you are on a daily trek to and from the hospital. Every day was the same day – a 30-minute drive, 20 minutes to find a parking space, then into the cancer care unit, down to the basement, pass all the sick people, radiotherapy running 15 minutes late, glass of water 30 minutes before appointment, into the toilet, enema up the bum. Twenty minutes later, back in the toilet, bowels empty, sitting in the waiting room, guess the cancer of my fellow patients, name called, into the cubicle, clothes off, knock on the door, into the treatment room, small talk with the radiographers, into position on the bed, everyone leaves the room. Alone with my thoughts, the machine whirrs back and forwards over my nether regions, nuking everything in its path, me imagining cancer cells being obliterated. Out the door, run to the toilet, a satisfying pee, two more before I get in the car, head home bursting for another one and back tomorrow.

Fuck Christmas this year.

The enemas weren't too bad initially, and the side effects of the treatment negligible. A bit of tiredness maybe, but that was it. In fact, the only highlight (well, maybe not a highlight), occurred after my third or fourth treatment. I ran out of the cubicle as usual, up the corridor and into the first available toilet. On my way out, there was a radiographer there to greet me. I presumed she had tried to catch me earlier but in my desperation for a pee I had shaken her off.

'Could you please come back and take a seat in the waiting room, Mr Ferris?'

She looked a bit too stony-faced for my liking. I could feel a flutter of panic hit my chest.

I followed them down the hall, past three breast cancers, a throat cancer and two prostate cancers. I took a seat as I spoke.

'Is everything OK?'

She didn't smile.

'I'm sure everything is absolutely fine.'

That wasn't enough to stop the fluttering.

'What's absolutely fine?'

She sat down beside me.

'Something has shown up on your scan. I am just getting your consultant to have a look at the images. When he comes back to me, I will let you know. I would like you to wait here until he responds to us. I'm sure it's nothing to worry about.'

With that she disappeared back into her office. Despite her words of reassurance, I found plenty to worry about in the hour that I waited. I worried about cancer spreading, new tumours, more treatments and dying before my time. That's a good list for anybody to worry about. Eventually the door opened again and she came and sat beside me. I could feel my stomach jump as she began to speak.

'I've spoken to your consultant. He has had a good look at the mass and he says he is happy for you to go home and it is nothing to be concerned about.'

I wasn't happy with the explanation.

'Did he say what he thought the mass was?'

She got up to leave.

'Oh yes. He says it's most probably a testicle.'

'A testicle?'

'Yes. It's quite common. Do you have a testicle that sometimes retracts into your abdomen?'

I did. It was doing it right at that moment.

'Err… yes. It does happen sometimes.'

A testicle with stage fright.

'Well, there you go then. Mystery solved and panic over.'

I stood up and thanked her, embarrassment overtaking fear, as me and my retracting testicle made our way along the corridor. By the time I got to the car, anger had replaced embarrassment. I was angry. Really angry. Angry at my useless retracting testicle. I was annoyed that something so innocuous could cause me so much worry. But that's the problem when you've been diagnosed with cancer. Or in my case heart disease and cancer. Nothing seems innocuous anymore. A chest pain feels like a heart attack, a headache the beginnings of a stroke, and a stray testicle showing up on a scan is a giant tumour. OK, 'giant' is pushing it, but you get the picture. When disease and illness enter your life, it becomes impossible to ever go back to the days before they raised their ugly heads. I suppose you just have to find a new way to be. I hadn't got to that point yet.

I climbed into my car. I slipped my hand inside my jeans and pushed my annoying testicle out of my abdomen and back into its sack. By the time I'd reached the payment barrier the bastard had made its way back up again. I was going to push it back down again. Then I stopped myself. *Bollox to it!*

CHAPTER 21

Misbehaving testicle aside, the first two weeks of my radiotherapy were pretty uneventful. Monotonous but uneventful. Once or twice, when they were running a little late, I had the very real fear that I might wet myself between the time it took from drinking my water to having the treatment. Thankfully I avoided that humiliation. The treatment had so little impact on me, that I began to wonder if the big expensive looking contraption I was placed in everyday was actually delivering any radiation into my body at all. I had taken time off work for the duration of my treatment and was feeling a little embarrassed and somewhat guilty that I felt perfectly fine. Then the tiredness came.

I don't know when I noticed it first. I just became aware sometime during the middle of the treatment that every time I sat on the sofa I was falling asleep. Driving any distance became a bit of an issue. I just felt drowsy every time I drove. I was back to pulling the car over on occasion, in order to have a quick nap to ensure the safety of other road users. But it wasn't just the tiredness that hit me. When I wasn't sleeping, or wishing I was sleeping, I could be found on my other favourite seat... the toilet seat. I don't know if it was the daily enemas or the treatment itself but my toilet habits gradually became more and more unpleasant. I was sore anyway from inserting daily enemas up my backside but what started as occasional loose stools developed into regular painful diarrhoea.

That's how I spent Christmas 2017. Sleeping on the sofa, sleeping in the car or sitting on the toilet. I suppose that's why I don't remember much else about that time. I do remember sitting in the hospital café a couple of days before the big day itself being entertained by the 30-strong choir that had taken up position behind me. They sang beautifully. I looked around. Everyone else seemed to be joining in with the spirit of it all. The choir serenaded us with all the old traditional carols. There were bells ringing and children singing. Santa Claus made an appearance and 'ho-ho-ho'd' his way around the café, passing out sweets and chocolate. I declined his offer. I could happily have done without the whole jolly show – spending the second Christmas in a row visiting the cancer care unit was a guaranteed festive-mood buster if ever there was one. There was just something about hearing joyous carols ringing out over a cancer care department that didn't sit well with me. It felt like fake happiness in a place where genuine happiness had long since left the building. It just didn't work for me.

What did work for me were the constant emails I was now receiving from my editor, Roddy Bloomfield. I was choosing the photographs, the dedication, the captions for the photos, and making last-minute corrections to the text of my book. I spent my days in the waiting room of the radiotherapy department immersed in the finishing touches to the book. It was a great escape from my reality. It wasn't fake happiness, it was real. If the carols in the cancer unit saddened me, making plans for my upcoming book publication transported me from the misery and uncertainty of where life had taken me. It brought me to a place of genuine hope for the future. A future where I would be free of cancer, wide awake, off the toilet and back in the land of the living.

Even though I knew that the upcoming publication would be something to cherish, I still didn't really know what to expect. I had never been down this road before. I didn't even know a road like this existed for someone like me. As I read it again and made my last-minute changes, I still had a nagging doubt that it simply wasn't good enough to be published. Maybe it had all been a huge mistake on the part of my publisher? Maybe Roddy had backed a dud this time? He certainly hadn't given me the impression he thought he had. If anything, he'd given me enormous confidence that I'd written something worth reading. I'd met Roddy during the summer. He was convinced I had written a really special book. We'd met over lunch in Covent Garden and, after spending 15 minutes in my company, he leaned across the table.

'My dear boy. I don't know where this lack of confidence comes from. I will say this to you just this once. You have written a wonderful and unique book. You should be very proud of it. I am convinced people will love it. I have no doubt whatsoever about that.'

When I was editing it in the radiotherapy department, and the doubts crept in, I focussed on Roddy's words and took my confidence from him. I thought about the number of books he'd edited and published in the past. It was well over a thousand. I was buoyed by his faith in mine. Nevertheless, I would only know objectively how good it actually was when it was out in the public domain for anyone to read and critique. That day was just around the corner, a thought that was both exhilarating and terrifying.

My daily radiotherapy sessions prevented me from travelling to London to meet Hodder and Stoughton publicist, Karen Geary. She very kindly agreed to travel to Newcastle for our meeting. I was nervous as I waited in Central Station for her to come through the turnstiles. This was a whole new world for me. It's one thing typing a manuscript at the kitchen table, but it is a whole other thing still to secure a publisher like Hodder and Stoughton, work with an editor like Roddy Bloomfield, and now to be having a meeting with a publicist. And not just any publicist either. Karen Geary was the director of publicity. I didn't really know what to expect when I stood in the crowded train station. I scanned the throng spilling through the turnstile. I looked left and right for her but couldn't see her anywhere. I swivelled my head again. Still no sign of her. Where was she? Maybe she had missed the train? Maybe she'd finally read the manuscript and made a U-turn?

'You must be Paul.'

I turned my gaze to the well-spoken voice in front of me. A kind smile greeted my terror.

'I'm Karen. Karen Geary. So very good to meet you.'

She held her hand out to shake mine. I took it, pulled her in, and kissed her awkwardly on the cheek.

Kissed her! Jesus Christ. Who kisses a complete stranger when she clearly has her hand out to shake hands?

She ignored my nerves.

'Very nice to meet you Karen. I'm glad you recognised me. I was starting to panic a little.'

She raised a copy of the book she was holding.

'It's easy when you have a book full of photographs with you.'

A book. My book. My actual book. In her hands. Right in front of me. Jesus.

She noticed me gawping at it.

'Oh... you won't have seen the manuscript in book form I suppose?'

She supposed right. The typo-riddled Word document that I'd sent off to my agent over a year before was now being held up in front of me as a book. *A bloody book. My bloody book!* She handed it to me. I could feel by heart thumping out of my jacket as I held it.

'This is only a sample. Not the finished book. These are the ones we send to the press pre-launch.'

I didn't care. I didn't care that it wasn't the finished book, or that it was just a sample. It was my book. My words. All 100,000 of them, squeezed into this tiny bundle in my hands.

'It feels good doesn't it, Paul?'

She was smiling at me as I held on tight to it.

I nodded.

'It feels amazing.'

She pointed out of the station.

'Shall we go and have a coffee and discuss how we are going to let the world know about it?'

I led her to the nearest café I could find. As we sat drinking our coffee exchanging small talk and pleasantries, my eyes were drawn again and again to this beautiful thing that sat in the middle of the table. *The Boy on the Shed, by Paul Ferris.* It was such a surreal experience that I struggled to hold a coherent conversation with her.

I wanted to grab it off the table, bring it to my nose and sniff it. Smell it to see if it smelled like the ones I use to read as a boy. There was a short but blissful time where my mother would come back from her weekly shopping at Wellworths armed with two presents for me; sweets and a book. One week it was *Robinson Crusoe*, the next week *Ivanhoe*, the week after that *Great Expectations*, and the next week *Gulliver's Travels*. I would wait patiently for her at the door, before dashing off to my bedroom with my stash. There I would stuff myself with the sweets and sniff the book. Something about the smell. I don't know what it was, but there was something about the smell of the words on the page that totally transfixed me. When I'd finally had enough of book sniffing, I'd then go on to devour the words on every page.

'You can't have finished it already!'

My mother would shake her head, but her smile told me that I would be getting another book with her next weekly shopping. The quality of my sweets plummeted when Wellworths started selling cheap family bags imported from eastern Europe, but the books always remained of the same standard. They were always classics. There obviously must have been some offer on with her shopping during that brief but brilliant period. I can't imagine my mother just deciding one day that her 11-year-old football-mad son needed a bit of *Wuthering Heights* to go with his cheap sweets. Whatever was the cause of it, her weekly gift instilled in me a lifelong love of books. I have an equally passionate commitment to avoiding poor quality confectionary.

'You haven't written that book. Have you?'

That's what I imagined my mother saying, expressing her disbelief and joy, if she were sitting in that café in Newcastle in December 2017. I would have loved to have seen her face when she saw a book with my name on the front of it. It would have been beyond her comprehension. It wasn't quite *Wuthering Heights* or *Great Expectations*. But it was a book. My book. I was still daydreaming about unforgettable books and forgettable sweets when Karen snapped me back into the present.

'I'm delighted to be leading the publicity for your book, Paul. It is an incredible read and I know people are going to love it. I knew it was a special book when I was reading it on the train and missed my stop. I think it has a chance of becoming a big book.'

I lifted my gaze from the book on the table and studied her. She had the look of someone who didn't waste words on idle compliments. There was something about her. She possessed a gravitas that gave me confidence I was sitting with the right person to give my book its best possible chance. Two hours after I'd first kissed her, I walked her to the train station. I kissed her again on both cheeks, a little less awkwardly than how I'd welcomed her to Newcastle. I got in my car and headed for the Freeman Hospital. I checked my jacket pocket to make sure I hadn't forgotten my enema. As I walked into the radiotherapy department, I pondered for a moment to think about the places this life can take us. Mine had just taken me from an excited conversation about the publication of my book and promises of national TV and radio appearances, to sticking a tube of laxative up my bum in readiness for my treatment, all in the space of two or three hours.

*　*　*

'What are you smiling about?'

Geraldine was peering over her glasses from the other side of the kitchen table.

'Me? Smiling? Are you sure?'

She laughed.

'Yes, I'm definitely sure. It's been a while since I saw one on your face, but you were definitely smiling.'

I turned my phone around so the screen faced her.

'That. That's what I'm smiling about.'

She leaned over and took the phone from me.

'What is it?'

I got up and moved around the table.

'What do you think it is?'

She squinted at the screen. Our eyesight had been deteriorating in unison over the past few years. We'd recently had our eyes tested and had been prescribed our first pairs of glasses on the same day.

'It looks like a book. It's a bit blurred though.'

I took the phone off her and flicked to the slightly clearer image.

'There. Try that one?'

She let out a yelp.

'It's your book. Wow. Why are the photos so blurry?'

The photos were so blurry because I had taken them furtively, like some dodgy private eye, while Karen had visited the toilet. The suspicious glance the café owner gave me as I did so, ensured I only captured two furry images, both of which were barely identifiable as a book. I could have just asked Karen if I could take a photo. But I didn't. I hadn't wanted her to see what I undoubtedly was, some sad bastard who was unbelievably excited to see his words laid out in front of him in a book, behaving as if I'd just written *Robinson Crusoe* or *Ivanhoe*. I suppose it could have been worse. I could've asked her if I could sniff her copy. I'm glad I'd done neither. Instead, I'd taken my blurry photos. I'd stared at them for the rest of the day; while waiting for my enema to work, while waiting for my radiotherapy, while preparing dinner, and while sitting at the kitchen table watching Geraldine tapping into her work laptop.

'I think this calls for a bottle of wine, don't you?'

She was on her feet at the fridge before I had time to say yes. She poured me a glass and hugged me tightly.

'I think it's amazing what you have done. You should be very proud of yourself. I can't wait to see the book in the shops and go to Ireland and see it there too? Can you imagine?'

She let go and sat back down.

'What's the matter? Where has the smile gone?'

I took a sip of the wine.

'It's nothing really. I agree it's brilliant. It really is. I just can't help thinking of crap sweets and *Gulliver's Travels*. It seems such a long time ago now, but I wish...'

She'd heard the story so many times. She was around the table and hugging my neck.

'Your mammy would have been so proud of you. You know that. That is not a reason to feel sad today. It's a reason to be happy. She wouldn't have believed it would be possible for you or anybody else she knew to write a book. Be proud for her. She would want that.'

I rubbed her hand and stared at the image on the phone.

I was looking forward to sniffing my book. I missed my mother desperately even 30 years after her death. I sipped my wine. It tasted delicious. I missed my mother, but she could keep her crap sweets. I had another drink and then raised my glass to her.

I thanked her for the books.

CHAPTER 22

The end of my radiotherapy treatment was a bit of an anti-climax. I don't know what I was anticipating exactly. Or how I was expecting to feel when the last appointment was over. For weeks I'd watched as others had completed theirs. I'd been envious of them not having to make the daily trek into the bowels of the hospital anymore. I'd always know when someone else had completed his or her treatment as that person would triumphantly ring the bell that hung next to the reception area. As they did so, I and all the other sick people, would clap and cheer loudly. It was as if the bell ringers had beaten cancer forever. They were on a fast-track back to life. The little poem written next to the bell said as much. Yet as I walked towards it on my way out of the radiotherapy department for the final time that really wasn't how I was feeling at all. I didn't feel like I was on the fast-track back to life. Yes, my unpleasant and destructive radiotherapy treatment was finished, but my cancer journey wasn't. I rang the bell anyway.

I felt a bit of a fraud as I accepted my round of applause from the pale woman in the headscarf and her worried husband. I was no more certain that day that I had beaten my cancer than I'd been on the day of my first session. How could I be? I'd have to wait three months to see my oncologist. It wasn't until that meeting that I would have any idea if the radiation had done the job the surgery hadn't. He would let me know if my PSA was back to being undetectable, or if my latest course of treatment had been in vain. Even then, if my PSA was undetectable, that would only give me respite for another three months until the next PSA test result. Then there was the hormone treatment I was still on. Its job was to dampen down the effects of the cancer. If it was doing its job as it should, then it would be masking the true blood PSA reading anyway.

I hated this new game I was playing with cancer. I was on the very treatment path I had rejected from the outset. I had dismissed it because it had provided me with no certainty. No definitive moment where I would be able to stand up and say, 'That's it. It has gone. I have beaten my cancer for good.' Only surgery had provided that tantalising prospect. Once my surgery had failed, however, I was forced into playing this alternative game with cancer that I hadn't wanted to play in the first place. In this new game, there would be no early victory for me. It was a game where I would never get that satisfaction of shouting from the rooftops, 'I have won. I have beaten cancer.' I would never have the real satisfaction of ringing that bell, and that truly meaning something to me. The whole point of opting for surgery was so that I could have my moment. So that I could one day gather my family around me, pull them in closely and tell them that my cancer was a thing of the past. I chose surgery so that one day in the future maybe on a visit to the pub or maybe when out for a meal with friends, I could casually throw in the old line: 'Oh the prostate cancer? Yeah, that's cured. It's in the past. It was a bit of a pain in the arse for a little while, but I'm done with it now.'

As I finished my radiotherapy, I didn't feel like I was done with it. I was still worried it wasn't done with me either. The physical evidence it wasn't done with me was with me every day. Even on days when I felt like I was making progress, the side effects of my various treatments would stop me in my tracks. Maybe I'd go a whole month without needing my incontinence pads. I'd be feeling good about myself and the future again. Normality would be returning to my life. Then something would come along and remind me that all was still utterly changed in my world.

I'd only been two weeks into my radiotherapy when one of those moments occurred. I was sitting in the car when I felt urine leaking out of me. It just seeped out. Despite my best clenching efforts, I was powerless to stop it. It was soul destroying. I had worked so hard since my surgery, to rid myself of that particular embarrassment, that I had no longer required pads. But it was back. It was just a tiny drop. Then the tiny drop became three tiny drops, four or five times a day. Tiny drops go a long way when they are leaking through your jeans. I doubled down on my pelvic floor exercises in the hope of once again stemming the flow and becoming dry once more. It proved a pointless pursuit. The tiny drops became a dribble, and the dribbles were happening any time, all the time. There was no doubt about it – my radiotherapy treatment had made me incontinent once more. So much so that by the time I was ringing my bell and taking the applause from my sparse audience, I was back to relying on my Tena For Men pads.

With Isla, I could live in the moment. She slept over at our house weekly. As soon as we heard her stirring, Geraldine would lift her from her cot and bring her into our bed. We'd lie for an hour or two just listening to our granddaughter laugh and play. I started to sing to her one day. She smiled so brightly that I haven't stopped singing to her since. I'd sing *My Girl, Sunshine on My Shoulders,* and some old Irish songs that my mother used to sing around the house – *I'll Tell My Ma* and *Believe Me, If All Those Endearing Young Charms* – I saw no harm in a bit of early brainwashing for her. Whatever the future holds for Isla and whether or not I'm a part of it, I will always have those moments with her, when she was too young to know how much she was loved. She will one day learn how much she helped her granda navigate his way through his most difficult period. I will cherish her forever for that.

My other great distraction from the cancer treatment and its hideous side effects, was the upcoming book launch. I'd been sent a publicity schedule which focussed heavily on the week of the launch. I was excited to see interviews scheduled for BBC Breakfast, Radio 2, TalkSPORT, Radio 5 Live, and local TV in Newcastle and in Northern Ireland. This was to be accompanied by impressive coverage in several national and local newspapers. Two days before publication, I sat with Karen in a brightly lit office at the BBC's studios in Salford. I thanked her for everything she had done. I told her that the publicity she had secured for *The Boy on the Shed* was way beyond anything I could ever have hoped for.

'Nonsense. No need to thank me. It's a brilliant book and no matter what happens with it, you should be really proud of it.'

I was grateful and encouraged by the support of someone who had clearly been on this path many times before with better and more successful authors than me.

Author! As I sat there with Karen, I felt unworthy of the title. By the time I made my way to the green room, I felt like a complete imposter. I walked to the room to be met by singer Michael Bolton. He greeted me enthusiastically, and very graciously asked me why I was there. I rambled on for two minutes about my story and the book and told him how nervous I was. He smiled and shook my hand. He told me just to repeat, on air, what I had said to him, as it sounded like a fascinating tale. He could well have just been being polite, but his words calmed my nerves. That calm didn't last long as one of the production team called my name. Another one started fussing around me. She put a microphone pack in my jacket pocket and a microphone on my lapel. My legs were now jelly. I followed her through a solid door. We skipped around a hundred cables and wires. We weaved through cameras. Finally, we emerged into the bright glare of the breakfast TV studio. The hosts, Dan Walker and Louise Minchin, were in dialogue with the producer as I slipped onto the chair next to them. Louise must have sensed me shaking next to her. She leaned over and spoke to me. She possessed a warm and friendly demeanour.

'Don't be nervous. You'll be fine. We will look after you.'

Her kindness had a settling effect on me. I watched the man behind the camera count down to the moment that I would be interviewed live on national television about a book I'd typed on two fingers with the expectation that maybe someday my kids might decide to read it. It was beyond my comprehension. It felt like it was happening to someone else, and I was just looking on. I felt like the interview went well. I don't think either of the presenters had read the book, not surprising, since they must get sent hundreds every year. But although they may not have read it, they had very obviously done their research. I really enjoyed the whole experience. Well, perhaps not quite all of it. Halfway through answering one of their questions, I felt a drop of urine – just a drop – make its way unimpeded past my last line of defence. I clenched everything I could clench, to stop myself from wetting my pants on national television. It was all in vain. I felt it leaving my body. I experienced a moment of panic before I remembered that I was back to wearing my trusty pads. The first drop was followed by a steady stream. Once I'd realised I was wearing my pad, I unclenched myself and let it flow. The rest of the interview passed in a wet blur. I had no real idea how it had gone until I got back to the small office where Karen met me with a beaming smile.

'Well done. That couldn't have gone any better.'

Instantly, messages started pinging on my phone from excited friends and family, and people I hadn't spoken to for years. They were all telling me how well I'd done. They were complimentary to the presenters for how well they'd handled the interview. Thankfully, no one, apart from me, was any the wiser that I had wet myself through the entire second half of it.

I walked with Karen towards the station. We had a coffee and a chat about the rest of the publicity she had lined up for me and my book. I was extremely grateful that the fate of my scribblings was in the hands of someone as professional as her. She really made me believe that the book was one of the best projects she'd worked on. As she sipped her coffee and answered her emails, I tried to think of the number of books that she must have worked on. Not only that, but also the quality of books that must have come across her desk. For her to be so buoyed by my amateurish efforts was something that I suddenly felt very proud of. She lifted her head from her screen.

'So just to confirm Paul. We have TalkSPORT, Radio 2, BBC 5 Live. Then we have BBC and ITV in the North East, ITV in Northern Ireland, RTE, BBC Radio Newcastle and BBC Radio Ulster. And beIN Sports in Dubai. Then there is the national press and local press here and in Northern Ireland also. I'm a bit disappointed I haven't been able to secure more coverage for you, but this is a great platform for publication in two days' time.'

Disappointed? Jesus! I'd have got less publicity for killing someone! If it were appropriate to do so I'd have reached over the table and kissed her again. The volume and quality of the publicity she had secured meant that at least my book would be widely read. If that was the case and people liked it, then they would tell their friends about it. If they hated it, then it would disappear into nothingness but at least she had given it an amazing chance. I left her at the station and headed for my train. My head was buzzing with the possibilities for the book. I found my seat on an overcrowded cabin and settled in to read the dozens of 'good luck' and 'well done' messages from earlier. I was about to put my phone away when I received an email from the publisher. It was from Fiona Rose, who'd helped edit the book and had done a great job with that task. There in bold, she'd copied a one-line message from an internal email sent to all staff at the publishers. It read:

After Paul Ferris's appearance on BBC Breakfast *this morning,* The Boy on the Shed *has risen to number 24 in Amazon Book Sales and to number 1 in Sports Biographies.*

I felt my pulse race and my chest pound as I read it again. I searched Amazon for the book and found it just where the message told me it would be. I sat transfixed staring at the screen. Thanks to the efforts of the Hodder team my book was going to have a chance. It was going to be read by a lot of people. The thought of a complete stranger reading my innermost thoughts and fears filled me with dread. It also filled me with incredible excitement. I was nervous that people wouldn't like the story, that it would bore them, but I was proud too. Proud, that my random scribbles existed in the world and would continue to exist long after I no longer did. I left my seat and pushed my way through the crowd. I slipped into the smelly bathroom and changed my pad. I bought some water and made my way back to my seat with my dry nappy firmly in place. I clicked on the Amazon page again. My book was number 24 on Amazon and number 1 in Sports Biographies. The train suddenly lurched to the right. My cup of water jumped off the table and onto my lap. I could only laugh. Nothing was going to spoil this day for me. Certainly not a drop of water seeping into my pad.

CHAPTER 23

Nothing was going to spoil the next few days either. I was determined to enjoy the book launch and vowed not to let the leaking parts of me, the dysfunctional parts of me, or the worried parts of me, get in the way of that. I just pushed all of them as far back into my head as they would go. The traumas of my past and my fears for the future were temporarily buried by my determination to enjoy every moment of the present. And it worked.

Incontinence pads aside, the next few days were probably the most rewarding of my life. I had played for Newcastle United at 16 and had been a physiotherapist there during an amazing period in the club's history. I'd gained a master's degree. I'd converted to law and became a barrister. I'd been part of Alan Shearer's management team, before helping build a business from nothing. They were all achievements I looked back on with quiet pride but writing a book and becoming a published author was just something that surpassed all of them, in my eyes. I don't know why. Maybe it was because it came along at a time when I really needed something positive in my life while dealing with my heart disease and prostate cancer. Or maybe it was because having a book published was something that stretched further than anything my boyhood imagination could conjure up. When I'd sat in a classroom at St Patrick's secondary school in Lisburn, having failed my 11-plus, shortly after the petrol bombing of my home, becoming a published author was simply beyond my horizon.

Whatever the reason I didn't care. I was just lost in the moment. I moved from bookshop to bookshop signing hundreds of copies.

I moved from TV studio to radio station, then on to interviews with national print media. I loved it, every second of it. Walking past a bookshop and watching a stranger pick up the book I had written, studying them as they scanned my work to establish if it was worth reading, was an uplifting experience. Watching him or her as they walked towards the counter and actually paid money for my writing was frankly mind-blowing.

At the end of my marathon promotional odyssey, I was invited to visit Northern Ireland for a final round of TV, radio and print media interviews. When they were done, I was scheduled to visit the two bookshops in the centre of my hometown, Lisburn. Eason's and Waterstones were situated in the main street of the town. The plan was for me to arrive unannounced and unheralded to sign their stock and hopefully aid sales. I was tired and hungry as I made my way from Market Square into Bow Street. I dragged my suitcase along the pedestrian walkway that was once the busy road of my childhood. An IRA car bomb had guaranteed no traffic would ever be allowed along there again. My increased incontinence since my radiotherapy meant that I was leaking like an old tap into my already sodden pad with every other step I took towards the bookshops.

As I pissed my way along Bow Street, I was struck by how derelict the once busy shopping hub of my childhood was. All the big stores were gone and had been replaced by charity shops, hairdressers' and empty units. The town centre had died some years ago, the result of having a rejuvenated Belfast just down the road, the closure of Thiepval Barracks and the subsequent redeployment of military families, and the arrival of an out-of-town shopping mall at Sprucefield. A couple of pensioners chatted to each other outside a bakery. A young woman carrying two heavy bags came towards me. She stopped to change her grip before hurrying on. Apart from that, the entire street was deserted.

Well, not quite. As I lifted my eyes beyond the weighed down woman, I could see signs of life in the direction I was heading. I searched for the bookshops. Eason's and Waterstones stand next to each other on the right-hand side of Bow Street as you walk from

Market Square. I wasn't quite sure what I was looking at when I saw the small crowd huddled in the distance. As I got closer, I could feel my heart jump a little. The crowd was gathered around the entrance to Waterstones. I allowed myself a moment to hope that they might be waiting for me. I dismissed it quickly and imagined someone had taken ill and the others were providing essential care, maybe. Or perhaps a scuffle had broken out and some peacemakers were dampening the fire? It wouldn't have been the first fight Bow Street had witnessed over the years, although admittedly the fights that had occurred before were unlikely to have flared up outside these bookshops. As I approached, I began to recognise some familiar faces in the crowd. Maybe they were here for me after all. As I reached the door of Waterstones, my brother Joseph emerged from the huddle. He opened his arms and hugged me.

'What kept you? It's packed in there and some of them aren't even our family!'

I looked at his smiling face.

'Really?'

He laughed and pushed me forward.

'Yes, really. There's been a sign in the window for the last few days announcing the prodigal son's return. Now get in there and don't keep them waiting.'

He was pushing me towards the door as I answered him.

'But it was supposed to be a private thing where I just come and sign stock?'

He laughed and pushed harder.

'Well, it's not too private now I can tell you.'

He took my suitcase from me and I took a deep breath. I could barely get through the door as I tried to step into the shop. It was jam-packed with familiar and unfamiliar faces. My family, extended family, old boyhood club managers, old friends and complete strangers all buzzed around me. Everywhere I looked someone was smiling at me. If they weren't doing that then they were shaking my hand. The excited shop manager introduced herself to me and ushered me to a chair next to a mountain of my books.

'We weren't quite expecting this many people. I hope you won't mind signing lots of books for them?'

Mind? I didn't mind. I really didn't mind. The next hour was one of the most brilliantly surreal moments of my life. Sitting in the middle of Waterstones bookstore in my hometown, signing copies of the book I had written many miles away in the solitude of our home in the north east of England was without doubt one of the most pleasurable experiences I've ever had. I don't know if it was because I had never expected to write a book that anyone would ever want to read. Or if it was simply a glorious interlude from the slog I was on with my prostate cancer. Or it may have been just the fact that I was back in Lisburn in these circumstances all those years after I'd left to pursue my dreams of being a footballer. This town used to frighten me so much when I was a boy. I had grown up here and witnessed all of its murderous sectarian hatred. I used to be too afraid to walk up Bow Street on dark nights. Some sickening beatings had occurred here during the bleakness of The Troubles. I had been a reluctant traveller, but I'd escaped to Newcastle with the promise of fame and glory to follow. I had carried my family's hopes and dreams with me. For a brief period, it had looked like I would succeed. But I hadn't succeeded. I had failed. I was too ashamed to return home after the end of my football career. The devastation of that failure and my mother's death soon afterwards ensured I was destined for a life in exile. Yet here I was, 37 years later, returning to Lisburn in triumph. Paul Ferris, failed footballer, was now Paul Ferris, published author. Maybe that was it? Maybe that's why that day felt so special to me? I really don't know. I only know that it did. Not even my saturated pad could spoil it.

The day wasn't entirely without hiccups. One by one they came to have their book signed and one by one they each had a story to tell. Of our shared childhoods, of when we last saw each other, of family members lost, or ailments lived with. One by one they hovered on my shoulder, talking for too long, oblivious to the sighs of the person behind who would come and do the same. I smiled and talked to all of them because I was genuinely excited to be there and grateful that they were there too. But there was one question I got asked repeatedly in that bookshop that came to fill me with dread. It may well be a universal question, but it feels to me like a uniquely Irish one. It is a simple question; a short question, but a cruel question to ask anyone. Yet still it was asked, again and again and again. It is designed to fill the recipient with utter dread.

You don't remember me, do you?

An awkward question at any time. But on days like this, when you are confronted with a hundred people, some of whom you haven't seen, heard or thought about for over 37 years, then it's brutal. I spent half my time in Waterstones frantically searching for names to put to faces that were often 35 years older than when I last saw them. I soon developed a strategy to get me through the day. It worked, mostly. In answer to every, 'You don't recognise me, do you?' or 'You have no idea who I am, do you?' I would just smile and lie through my teeth. 'Of course I recognise you. I certainly do remember you. I have every idea who you are. I remember you only too well. How's the family? I hope life has been kind to you. It certainly looks like it has. You are looking brilliant. You look great. Now, who am I signing the book to?'

I'd found my strategy. I'd cracked it. 'Who am I signing the book to?' A great question. They had to give me their name, or at least the family member's name, I was signing the book for. That then gave me another chance to identify them or bluff a bit more about the family member until they left. Job done.

I was settling nicely into my lying, and getting near to the end of the queue, when a big man smelling of alcohol and fried food leaned into my face with the all too familiar question.

'Great to see you Ferrie.' My unfortunate boyhood nickname.

'Jesus, Paul. It must be nearly 40 years since I last saw you. You're looking great, so you are.'

He was a better liar than me! He pushed his copy of my book onto the table in front of me and asked the dreaded question.

'You haven't a fucking clue who I am, do you wee man?'

I turned to face his breath and caught sight of some stray egg that had escaped his mouth and partially hidden itself in his wiry beard. I searched his ruddy features for anything I could hang my hat on. Looked into his sunken red eyes. I had nothing. Not a flicker of recognition. I lied my way forward.

'Don't be so daft. Of course I recognise you. How could anybody forget that face?'

I'd bought myself time. I wasn't giving up that easily. Besides, I had my own killer question, that was guaranteed to achieve the desired results when all else had failed. I opened his book, readied my pen, and turned to his eggy chins.

'Who am I signing it to?'

Got him.

'Just sign it to me.'

Shit! Think!

'How are you spelling that?'

He had nowhere to go.

He spelled his name slowly as I triumphantly wrote it down. 'P... A... U... L'

I didn't look up at him, or his egg, as he left with a weary pat on my lying back. I suppose even the best strategies have their flaws in the end.

A family dinner in a local restaurant was followed by too many drinks back at Denise and Kieran's house. Their home had become my second home on my visits to Ireland over the years. As I sat in their kitchen surrounded by the happy faces of their grown-up kids, my mind drifted to those days when I was a boy sitting with my own mother in our tiny kitchen in Manor Park. I know she had many hopes and dreams for me, most of them involving me hitting dizzying heights as a world-famous footballer. That dream died just before she did. As the effects of the wine kicked in, I wished more than anything that she could have shared this dream too. Her son was a published Author. I hadn't really felt like an Author. Not until today. Not until I saw my book on the big table in Waterstones and signed one after the other for the people I had pretended to remember. I was still wallowing in my glory as I made my way into the spare bedroom. I crashed fully clothed, on top of the bed. Nothing could spoil my bliss. I was an author. A published author. Now I just had to hope people would read it and hopefully enjoy it.

I awoke in the darkness and squinted at the red glow of the digital clock lighting up the corner of the room. I searched for my phone and typed in the book title. I clicked the Amazon link for biographies, just to look at my newly published book, to make sure it all wasn't just a dream. The book cover image flashed up. Me, as a boy, stared back at me, the middle-aged drunk man. *The Boy on the Shed* sat proudly at number 1 in Sports Biographies. I was about to flick the phone off when I caught sight of the reviews section. I had one review already, less than one full day since publication. *Brilliant. Somebody was keen. He or she must have bought it on release, then devoured every page, before hurriedly posting his or her five-star opinions for the world to see.* What a great and unexpected start to my new life as an author. I sat up and fumbled for my glasses. I wanted to savour the moment, my first review. And there it was: 'Two stars – disappointing.'

Bollox!

I might well have been a published author but if my reviews were going to be 'two stars – disappointing' then I was obviously going to be a not-very-good published author. I threw the phone on the floor, pulled my clothes off and climbed under the covers. I tried and failed to get back to sleep. Two stars! My book felt better than that.

CHAPTER 24

'He's biased.'

Denise sat the mug of tea in front of me as she spoke.

'Who's biased?'

I brought the steaming cup to my mouth, burned my lips, and quickly lowered it on to her kitchen table. The smell of the bacon sizzling had me wishing I wasn't back to following my vegan diet. These were the hardest days. The hangover days. Ordinarily, I didn't even think of the deprivation my new lifestyle entailed. The fear of having another heart attack, which might kill me, was a good motivator. I hoped my new diet would be able to stop the disease that had taken my mother's life far too soon from taking mine also. It empowered me to think that maybe heart disease wouldn't get me after all. Those thoughts were usually more than enough to ensure I persevered with my new way of life. I mostly didn't even miss my former meat-filled life. Except on hangover days. Hangover days were different. On hangover days bacon smelled better than it ever had before. Pizza looked cheesier, fish and chips smelled fishier, chocolate screamed at me from every shop window. Not to mention the steak, ham and eggs that tried to sneak their way into my supermarket trolley and then into my clogged arteries. On hangover days, images of Colonel Sanders' bearded face would regularly invade my head. I wouldn't care but I didn't even miss his secret recipe chicken on hangover-free days.

The only times I ever came close to breaking my vegan diet were on those long days that followed the night-before's drinking. And the night before today had been a good one. No. Not a good one. A bloody great one. Apart from the two-star review reminding me that I was a shit author.

'There, look.'

I squinted at Denise's phone. I could make out the blurred review.

'Yeah, I saw it. What if the book is shit? How embarrassing. It's out there now and I can't take it back. This is going to be really uncomfortable. The details of my life are out there, and people are laughing at it. Jesus, what was I thinking writing the thing in the first place?'

Denise was undaunted.

'Shut up you idiot. The book is brilliant. I've read it. It is going to be fantastic. People will love it.'

She tapped on her phone.

'There you go. He's biased. I told you. Have a read of that.'

On her screen were the details of the reviewer. A local councillor in Northern Ireland. A TUV Councillor. The name meant nothing to me.

'What's the TUV?'

Denise raised her eyes like she was trying to pull the answer down from the top of her head.

'Ah... let me think. Ah, it's the Traditional Unionist Voice. It's more right-wing than the DUP. The TUV thinks the DUP has gone soft.'

I had a quick scroll through the TUV manifesto. It was like stepping back in time, to before the Good Friday Agreement had brought much needed peace, enlightenment and understanding to Northern Ireland. The manifesto was the politics of division, entitlement and one-eyed sectarian bilge. It was a type of politics that I had always despised. I'd hoped it had been consigned to history, along with the dinosaurs who'd propagated it. I'd always had my doubts though and those doubts were confirmed as I scrolled the page. When I'd finished digesting the hate-filled bile in front of me, she took the phone from me and flicked to the Amazon page.

'Have a read of the review again, now that you know it was written by someone with that political outlook.'

She was right. When I read it again, I laughed out loud. It was all I could do. The reviewer, who had been captivated by my writing, was nevertheless disappointed that I hadn't mentioned IRA violence in the book. He was annoyed that I'd only concentrated my writing on my very real fears and experiences of UDA/UVF violence. Yet, that genuine terror had blighted my childhood, as an innocent Catholic boy growing up in the staunchly Protestant stronghold of Lisburn. He was further concerned that I should stop living in the bitterness of the past and he hoped that one day I would be able to dispel the hurt. He was a member of a political party that lived firmly in the past! He finished his review by claiming to have met me and wishing me well for the future. I was still shaking my head when I passed her the phone.

'Jesus Christ. He's disappointed we weren't subjected to IRA violence as well. Has he not realised that I could only write about loyalist violence because that was the violence that was perpetrated against our family? It's not a competition. He says he has met me. He must have had to hold his nose when he did.'

I wasn't done. I was disgusted.

'You keep telling me this place has changed, but it'll take generations for that sort of crap to stop, if it ever will. That's why I am glad I don't live here anymore and don't have to put up with it. It would drive me insane to have to deal with that nonsense every day.'

Denise shook her head.

'It has changed. People are no longer killing each other. We're no longer frightened to have a party in our kitchen in case somebody throws something through the window. It has changed. We can go anywhere we want for a drink in the town now. Mind you, there are three of four places I still wouldn't go…'

I didn't let her finish.

'There you go. You don't even realise what you've just said.'

She shrugged.

'What have I said?'

'You've just admitted that this place is still the same. Still full of hate. Still full of fear. There are three or four places you don't feel comfortable going. Christ, it's 2018, The Troubles have been over for more than 20 years, and you still don't feel comfortable drinking and eating in the town you were born in and have lived in all of your life. I wrote a book, and some right-wing prat rushes to read it, and then posts a review within 12 hours of its publication, criticising me for not highlighting IRA atrocities. I didn't directly experience any IRA violence. If I had, then I'd have written about it. The only violence I was subjected to was the violence I wrote about. Must I not write about evil, when that evil ruined my childhood? Or only write about evil when it serves a political agenda? This place makes me sick sometimes. Where are the voices of reason? Of love? Of harmony? I'll tell you where. They're silenced by the louder ones of tribalism, bigotry and hate. In this place, they always will be sadly. Murder is murder, no matter who commits it. Fear is fear, no matter who feels it. It's not that difficult to grasp is it?'

Denise poured some hot water into my cooled tea.

'Have you finished?'

'Yes.'

'Good. Cos you have another review.'

I took the phone from her. I read the five-star review with a mixture of pride and relief. I checked to make sure it wasn't one from an enthusiastic family member and that it was from an actual person who'd genuinely enjoyed my writing. When I was satisfied it was, and just as the fried breakfasts were making their way onto the table, I took a copy of my book and slipped out of the house.

The rain spat at me as I made the short but familiar trek. It was one I made every time I visited my hometown. I tucked my book inside my coat, and nodded at a couple of familiar, wizened faces en route. I climbed the steps and made my way past the uniform rows until I found myself in my usual place. I stared at the writing on the heart-shaped stone. It read: *In loving memory of Theresa Corrigan*. I'd first visited this grave when I was six years old. Theresa was my maternal grandmother, who had died in 1971. I remember standing at the end of her bed as she lay in our sitting room. She called my name. When she was sure I was paying attention, she made me solemnly promise not to cry for her when she was gone. In the weeks that followed her death I disobeyed her every night. The kind presence who'd brought me sweets every day was gone. She had looked after me as an infant in the days when my mother was still well enough to work. And although she did scald me with tomato soup once, her tears told me she hadn't meant to. One day this giant presence in my life was there and the next day she was gone. She disappeared the same year my mother had her first heart attack. 1971 wasn't a great year on reflection. Back then my religious belief was strong and my mind had not yet opened to questioning its dogma. I prayed to my dead grandmother every night, and every day after school I would come to this spot where I had watched her being lowered into a hole in the ground, which was now covered with the beautiful heart-shaped headstone. I would just sit there and tell her about my day. Most of my prayers to her were begging her not to ask for my mother to follow her too soon. She granted my wish for a few years until in 1987, I watched bereft as her daughter Bernadette was lowered gently into the cold earth on top of her mother.

Bernadette had threatened to do it for years. Heart attack after heart attack ensured that when my mother finally joined her mother it was no real surprise to anyone. That inevitable outcome in no way eased the pain or prevented her death from opening a gaping hole in my heart. Below my mother's name on the gravestone was that of my father Patrick, who died in 1999. I think death came as a relief to him. Too often, I witnessed him lost when sitting in a room full of people. I'd felt his loneliness, as he changed into his suit beside me on my wedding day. I would often glimpse the sadness in his eyes as he was surrounded by the love and joy of his grandchildren. To bear witness to that was to understand the love that had gone before and the loss that he now felt. My father was a shell of himself in the years that followed my mother's passing. So much so, that I don't doubt he asked his God every night to take him to her. The day he died, he believed with every fibre of his being that that is where he was going. I still envy him that certainty. In 2004, my brother Patsy joined them in this final resting place. His troubled soul buried with his parents.

My brother Eamon's still-born child was also laid here with the family she never got to meet.

As I stood, with my book in my hand, staring at their names on the gravestone, I felt my eyes fill. I wiped a tear that was mingling with the rain, before another made its way out and landed onto the cover of the book. I tried to stop the next one, but the one after that was pushing it further down my cheek. Then I gave up. I stood there by my parents' grave with my book in my hand and I wept like a baby. I wept for the loss of them, for the time we would never share again. I wept for the certainty they'd possessed that we would be reunited in death. I wept for my own certainty that we wouldn't. They were gone forever. Gone from this earth, never to return, never to laugh or cry, never to feel or touch. Never to hug me and say well done on the publication of your book. Never to say I'm glad you married Geraldine or look how your boys have grown or ask if I'd like a cup of tea. I wept for all of it.

I was still weeping when I heard a voice. I looked up towards the path. There was an old man propping himself up on a zimmer frame. He was shouting in a whisper at me and waving his hand. I peered at him through my red eyes. I needed to wipe my nose, which was delivering a steady stream of salty mucous into my mouth. I resisted the temptation. I didn't want to draw attention to the fact that I had been uncontrollably crying over the grave of people who had been dead for 40, 30 and 20 years respectively. He shouted at me again.

'You don't recognise me, do you?'

I felt the familiar pang of dread from my book signing.

He laughed.

'Jesus, Ferrie. You don't recognise me at all do you boy?'

I strained from 20 yards through bloodshot eyes to see I if could place the young man somewhere inside the old one. It was a futile pursuit.

He was enjoying himself now.

'Go on. Have a go. Who am I?'

I thought about shouting, 'Well if you don't know. How am I supposed to know?' I didn't. I was worried he wouldn't get the joke.

What is it with people? Why do they feel the need to ask other people whether or not they remember them after 40 years of not seeing each other? After 40 years, I can hardly remember my own name, never mind theirs. I stared at him. He stared at me. I couldn't even have a stab at it.

'I'm sorry. You've got me. It's been a long time.'

He shook his head in mock disappointment.

'It's me. Mousey Martin.'

Mousey Martin? From Manor Park?

Everybody on my estate had a stupid nickname. Mousey Martin, Fogey Fagan, Petsee McKee, Pip Corkin. Ferrie wasn't such an imaginative one. Fogey's brother, Micky, had the best one, Gedabit, because if he ever saw you with sweets or anything edible in your hand, he would always ask for some. He struggled a little with his pronunciations back then, so his 'give me a bit' became 'gedabit'. A far superior nickname to Ferrie.

Mousey Martin was one of the boys who was a little older than me. He'd always been kind to me, and it was sad to see him so physically frail. As I studied this gaunt figure in front of me, I thought about how, as the years skip past, this life is brutal on all of us. My heart attack and prostate cancer were testament to that. We chatted for a short while about his physical ailments, football, the book and my family. I stood and watched as he shuffled through the gates of the graveyard. I let my mind wander to days on the estate. We'd play football, hide and seek, and cards. Or we'd just hang around on the corner being children pretending to be adults. I'd play out all day and dread the moment when my mother would call me in for bed. I watched Mousey disappear and looked back at the grave. I conjured an image in my mind of Manor Park on a summer's day. We were playing 15-a-side football with our shirts for goalposts. My heart was thumping as I rode the tackles of the older boys. My head was spinning as I turned to celebrate another goal against Mousey and the big boys. Forty-five years later standing there at my parents' grave I attempted to steal back that moment. To reverse the punishing passage of time. I tried to steal back my childhood. The sunshine, the innocence, the happiness. I grabbed it for a brief second. Then it slipped tantalisingly out of my grasp. It always did and it always will. There is no going back. Only forward. The past is gone. I miss it sometimes. I said goodbye to my dead parents. My eyes and the rain poured over my book as I left the graveyard.

CHAPTER 25

In the weeks and months after the book launch my diary was filled with blood tests, and appointments with the oncologist and cardiologist. Their presence in my calendar meant that any enjoyment I was getting from the brilliant reviews for *The Boy on the Shed* were offset by a genuine fear for my future. When I was a child growing up in Ireland, then becoming a man playing professional football at Newcastle United, the thought that I would suffer a heart attack and have cancer before I was 52 would have been way beyond the realms of any imagination I was capable of. But here I was. The arrival of Isla and the early success of the book were welcome distractions. They couldn't, however, rid me of my despair at the hand my genes had dealt me. The untimely heart attack was one thing. The cancer diagnosis another. But both within three years of each other? That just felt wrong to me. I had a loving wife who'd been by my side since we were children. I had three amazing kids who were growing into equally great adults. My beautiful granddaughter made me smile and burst with joy every time I set eyes on her. My work at Speedflex was rewarding and beginning to bear real fruit after many years of struggle. The response to the publication of my book filled me with pride and satisfaction. But all of it meant nothing to me when I allowed fear to get in.

I fought against it, but when the fear sneaked in, it often caught me off guard. Its effects were soul crushing. I was usually able to fight it off at the first sign of my mood dropping. I would take the family out for dinner, book a break away, throw myself into my work or just play with Isla. There's something magical about watching a child just live and laugh in the moment. So I would join in with her. Sing songs to her, hold her close to me and tell myself all was well in my world. But it wasn't. Heart disease and cancer were my new life companions, and they weren't easy friends to part with. They were with me when I lay my head on the pillow at night and they were still there when I lifted it off the following morning. They were with me when I met someone new. They were with me when I met an old friend and we chatted about how life was treating us. They were most certainly with me on those days when I had to pay my regular visit to the GP to have my blood checked for my upcoming appointments.

The cardiology tests were usually straightforward. I had been back on my statin medication for a while. Their effects, coupled with my lifestyle changes, meant my cholesterol levels were always extremely low, so the likelihood of another heart attack was significantly reduced. That combined effort was going really well right up until the point that my muscles and joints began to ache so much that I could barely turn over in bed. That meant only one thing – I was once again having a reaction to my statins. My doctor had taken me off them at my last appointment and matters had improved considerably. My next blood test was to see if my cholesterol had risen as a result. If I couldn't tolerate my medication that was one thing. If I couldn't tolerate my medication and my cholesterol levels spiked, then that was an entirely different matter. Good cholesterol levels but intolerable muscle and joint pain, or no muscle and joint pain, but dangerously high cholesterol. I would still have a choice. It would just be Hobson's.

The PSA test was of much more pressing concern for me. I was due my first blood test result since undergoing my radiotherapy and hormone treatments. I was anxious and apprehensive when I called to the GP practice to retrieve them. I'd had the 'false positive' conversation with his receptionist previously. I'd intended to leave the results this time until my appointment with Dr Frew, but I needed to know whether or not my radiotherapy had worked. That curiosity had triumphed. I was now waiting patiently on the phone once more for a busy receptionist to deliver my results.

'Your PSA is 0.03 and the doctor is happy with it.'

She was desperate to get me off the phone again. My loosening bowels and cold sweat wouldn't allow her. I'd been down this road before.

'I'm sorry. Did you say my PSA was 0.03?'

'That's correct.'

I could feel my stomach jump. A reading of 0.03 meant my PSA was still detectable. It was exactly the same as it had been after my surgery. That was why I'd had to undergo further treatment in the first place. My PSA needed to be less than 0.03. Anything other than less than 0.03 spelled catastrophe for me. Any other reading signalled one thing only – my radiotherapy and hormone treatment hadn't worked. The obliteration of the nerves to my penis, the return of my incontinence, the enemas, the diarrhoea, the new breasts and tiredness would all be for nothing. The cancer was still there. I took a deep breath.

'I'm really sorry to be a pain, but could you look at it again and tell me if there is a sign or a symbol in front of the 0.03?'

I could hear her pressing buttons on her keypad.

'Let me see. PSA… PSA… PSA.'

My cancer… my future… my life.

'Yes. There is an arrow in front of the 0.03.'

'Could you tell me which way the point is facing?'

'Sorry?'

'The arrow. Which way is the point of the arrow facing?'

'Point… point… point.'

Cancer… future… life.

'Got it. It's pointing away from the first zero.'

My stomach settled.

'Are you sure? Are you sure it is pointing away?'

'Absolutely. I'm looking right at it. There are two lines moving into a point away from the number.'

<0.03! Less than 0.03! My cancer was undetectable!

I thanked her and hung up. I slumped in my chair. *My cancer was undetectable.* I made an unbreakable promise to myself that day. No matter how curious or desperate I was to find out the results of my blood test, I would never again call the GP reception desk for them. In future, I would wait until I was sitting in front of the oncologist. My fragile heart just wasn't up to the stress of it. Luckily, I was soon in front of my oncologist and Dr Frew greeted me with a smile and a firm handshake.

'You're in just the position we were hoping for at this stage, Paul. Your PSA is undetectable and long may that continue.'

I felt a surge of relief and a pang of fear.

'Does that mean you feel the radiotherapy has worked and it has likely got all the cancer that the surgery didn't?'

He rubbed his hand over his hair.

'Well, I would love to say yes, we have got it all and that it's never coming back, but I'm afraid I just can't say that. It's early days and you have just finished hormone treatment which can sometimes mask the results a little. So the best course of action is just to test your bloods every three months. The longer it stays undetectable, then the better that is.'

He must have read my face before continuing.

'This is nothing to be disappointed about. On the contrary…'

I interrupted him.

'Yes. I know. But what if the next test comes back and the PSA has risen?'

He leaned back in his chair and placed his hands behind his head.

'Then we will deal with that scenario should it ever arise. But please, rest assured that should that set of circumstances occur, then we have much more in our armoury than we have ever had before.'

I was more encouraged by that but not totally satisfied. I needed more.

'So if my cancer comes back, am I on a short, medium or long haul with it?'

He grinned at the question he'd probably been asked every day of his working life.

'If it comes back, and remember it may not, then you are still on a long haul with this. Everyone's cancer behaves differently. In your case, I would say you are in for the long haul with it. You should look at this as a marathon and not a sprint.'

That was good enough for me. With my fears sufficiently dampened I got up to leave. He spoke as I was at the door.

'How are you coping in general?'

The question caught me off guard. Before I had time to think I was telling him about my low moods, my new moobs, my leaky tubes, my lost libido and missing erections. I'm sure he wished he hadn't asked, but he ushered me back into my chair. He started typing into his desktop.

'Do you want to consider surgery to have your breasts reduced?'

I instinctively reached for my two new friends.

'Christ, they're not that big are they?'

'No. No. Not at all. It's just some men are so self-conscious after the hormone treatment that they choose that route. I'm just saying it's an option for you.'

It took me half a second to inform him that I wouldn't be taking the breast reduction route. I'd learn to live with my bra-worthy breasts. He moved on.

'I can refer you to someone you can talk to about your low moods if they're impacting on your wellbeing?'

I wanted to say 'yes' to that. But found myself brushing it off as if it was nothing to be concerned about. I have no idea why I chose to do that. Embarrassment maybe, fear of him thinking I was weak, not wanting to face the reality of the situation. I really don't know why I said all was fine. All was not fine. The mental challenges of dealing with the cancer and some of the hideous side effects from my treatments were slowly strangling my zest for life and crushing my hopes for the future. When my mood dipped it impacted on how I interacted at work and at home. Some days I would be so flat I didn't want to leave my bed. Other days I would be so angry that those close to me wished I hadn't left my bed. I was in a mental battle that I was clearly losing and yet couldn't find the courage to ask for help or put a name on it. I was angry at myself for not telling the truth. For my cowardice.

He even gave me a second chance.

'You're sure you don't want me to refer you to someone?'

'No. I'm fine. It's just a lot to deal with, but I'm fine.'

Those two small words. I was using them again. Two small words in the English language that mask a mountain of pain and paint a masterpiece of a lie. *I'm fine.* I wasn't fine then, and I haven't been fine on many occasions since. I even find it difficult to write, 'I'm not fine,' on a page. How strange that I should struggle so much to admit that to myself, or to a concerned friend or, in this case, to a caring doctor who might actually be able to help me?

The plain truth was that since my heart attack, and subsequent cancer diagnosis, my whole world view had shifted on its axis. Things I once enjoyed I no longer did. Places I once longed to visit no longer held their lustre. Conversations I loved having with friends now seemed meaningless. Days blended into weeks and seeped into months, and I failed to see the point of any of it. Now if that wasn't a job for a good counsellor then I don't know what was. Christ, I suspect even a bad counsellor could have a good go at that lot.

Despite that, I declined his offer of help in that department. Instead, I left his office with instructions to redouble my efforts with my pelvic floor exercises and his assurance that that would do the trick for my leaky tubes. I didn't get much help on the loss of libido side of things, just a knowing nod from him that the hormone treatment was the cause of that. I did secure an appointment with a urologist with a view to being fitted with a bionic penis! OK, so bionic penis was stretching it a bit, but I was going to talk to someone about penile implants so that I could once again have erections, albeit shrunken ones, without having the libido to give me the desire to have erections in the first place. Then with my new erections, I could have an orgasm, minus a prostate, that felt nothing like an orgasm with a prostate. If you can imagine having an orgasm that occurs without any of the build-up, anticipation and explosive release that an ejaculation of semen produces, then you are pretty much in the domain of the prostate-less orgasm. Not only that, the orgasm itself arrives like it's been dampened down to about a third of its intensity and you produce nothing. I'd spoken to Geraldine about it. The thought of having any kind of an erection when I orgasmed still seemed better that what I had at the minute, which was all of the above but without the scaffolding to hold my sorry bits in place. Is it any wonder I was a bit depressed?

CHAPTER 26

An upcoming court appearance, in the summer of 2018, was a reminder that the world hadn't stopped just because I was feeling sorry for myself, or couldn't shake off my latest low mood. I'd been visited by a detective five months before in relation to a case that was now being heard at Newcastle Crown Court. As I searched out my best suit for the day, or should I say, the only suit that fitted my expanding frame, I felt a shudder at just how close I may have come to being one of the victims seeking justice that day for the abhorrent sexual abuse they had suffered at the evil hands of the defendant, George Ormond. Instead, I was in the more fortunate position of being called as a prosecution witness. My evidence would hopefully help get justice for some of his innocent victims. It might bring some closure for one or two of the brave 18 men who'd had the courage to come forward and give evidence of their abuse as boys and their subsequent torment as adults.

They'd all suffered at the hands of a man I'd first encountered when I was an impressionable, shy 16-year-old. I'd met Ormond within days of my arrival at Newcastle United from my home in Northern Ireland in the autumn of 1981. He was also someone I would go on to work alongside, in the mid-1990s, when I was employed at the club as a physiotherapist. I was in court because of a conversation with an old friend that at the time had shaken me to the core. It had also led to me scratching around, out of my depth, trying to do the right thing.

Sometime in early 1997, Derek Bell rang me and asked if I'd meet with him for a drink. The call itself was a surprise because we had lost touch with each other over the years. We had once been great friends. Derek and his family had been a vital lifeline for me when I was a desperately homesick Irish boy, trying to find my way in my new world of professional football, my new city of Newcastle-upon-Tyne, and my new country of residence, England. Within weeks of my arrival at the club, Derek became my firm friend. He was a confident, handsome, talented and outgoing boy and was clearly one of the most popular boys in the group. He was also being groomed for bigger things by the coaching staff. He took me under his wing and invited me into his home. Every Thursday I would go and have tea there and most times I would sleep over. I'd share his bedroom, where we would lie on two single beds, talking about our girlfriends and our hopes and dreams of footballing greatness. The house was friendly and inviting. His mother and father would be there and his brother, Alan, was a permanent fixture, too. There was also one other individual who never missed a Thursday there. That person was George Ormond.

Ormond had been Derek's boys' club manager at Montague Boys Club, one of the great local teams that had produced several players who had gone on to have brilliant football careers at the highest level. Ormond now worked with Newcastle United's youth team. He was always around the football club. He was there in his coaching kit when I made my first appearance for the under-18 team shortly after my arrival at the club. I wasn't sure what his role was. The way he carried himself and spoke to me suggested that he was someone of influence who I had to impress if I hoped to make it in the professional game.

He clearly had a special relationship with Derek and his family. I was able to relax more in Ormond's company when he was in Derek's house on those Thursday visits. Derek turned 18 in the December after my arrival at the club. Ormond was 28. They booked a lads' holiday to Cyprus for the following summer and asked me to join them. I was so desperate to get home to Ireland and to Geraldine that I politely declined, so they holidayed as a pair, two best mates on a drinking holiday.

In the May before they travelled, I shared an experience with Derek that neither of us would ever forget. We made our debuts for the first team on the same day. Derek started the game against Blackburn, and I came on as a late substitute for Chris Waddle. We lost the game heavily, but both made the headlines – Derek for his assured performance in midfield, and me because, at 16 years and 294 days, I was the youngest player ever to play for Newcastle United. It was a glorious day for us both. Two young dreamers realising our dreams.

Professional football is a brutally cruel game and it dealt us both a bitter blow in the end. A knee injury shattered Derek's dreams after a handful of appearances. I fared a little better but succumbed to the same fate after a few more appearances. I had experienced the added joy of scoring a goal at St James' Park, which I still treasure to this day. Derek left the club three years before I did. We remained friends during that time but saw each other less often. When my career ended his mother took me in until I was able to find my feet again. As the years passed, we saw less of each other until finally we stopped communicating altogether. I had gone to university and found my way back to Newcastle United as a physiotherapist. Derek had taken a job working for the city council. We had both married and had children. We never fell out, just drifted away from each other.

In 1997, when he called me, it had been so long since we'd spoken that I didn't recognise the number in my phone. When I met him in my local pub a few days later, I barely recognised the man before me. His handsome youthfulness had been replaced by heavy jowls. His once narrow waistline, like my own, had been traded in for a more comfortable model. His eyes now sat sunken in deep sockets. I looked into them when we shook hands and he looked back into mine. He smiled but his eyes didn't join in. He glanced at me but quickly averted his gaze to the floor. As I brought our drinks to the small table in the middle of the near-deserted village pub it was clear all was not well with him. He shifted constantly in his chair. His eyes darted from me, to the table, then to the TV screen that was humming quietly in the background. I'd barely sat down when he grabbed me firmly by the arm, spilling my drink in the process. He was still holding my arm when he began to speak. I struggled at first to make sense of what he was saying, it was like he was speaking a foreign language. He was talking fast, almost whispering. He was glancing around the empty pub as if it was packed to the rafters with eavesdroppers, listening intently to the information he was imparting. It got so bad that he had me glancing around too. I took his hand off my arm and sat my drink down.

'You'll have to speak a bit louder and a little slower Derek. I can't understand what you are saying.'

He leaned in and spoke more clearly.

'Sorry mate. Sorry. Sorry. I was saying, that you need to get George out of the club. He's still working at the club and he shouldn't be there. Trust me. You need to get him out. That's all I'm saying. Just get him out.'

'George? George Ormond?'

'Yes. You need to get him out. I can't say anymore. He needs to go.'

I was more than a little confused at this point. George had been his great friend and as far as I was aware they were still friends.

'I thought George was a mate of yours. Anyway, he works with the youth team. I don't really have anything to do with him or his employment at the club. What's the problem?'

He was leaning into my face now. His eyes dancing and his body shaking.

'Problem? Oh, there is a problem alright. Big problem. You need to get him out.'

He sat back and took a swig of his beer. We sat in silence. I stared at the TV and waited for him to continue. He took so long to speak again that at one point I thought he wasn't going to bother. Then he leaned in again.

'What I'm about to tell you, I haven't told another soul. You need to promise it stays between us. OK?'

He had hold of my arm again. He was squeezing down hard. I nodded and he began to speak. His voice was quiet and his heightened emotional state evident.

'George abused me. He abused me from when I was 12 years old at Montague. Think of the worst sexual abuse you can imagine. He did that to me. Over many years. The abuse, and keeping it hidden from the world have destroyed my life. I was ashamed to tell anyone in case they thought it was somehow my fault. But now I know that I was groomed. From a very young age. He infiltrated my family and ingratiated himself with my parents to such an extent that it became impossible for me to find a way out. It started at the boys' club, then in car parks on the way home from training. Then in my home while my parents slept in the next room. I've carried the secret my whole life. It's cost me my marriage, my home and my family. I've been in institutions, where I have been sectioned, and I've tried to kill myself more than once. He's a fucking monster. You have to get him out of the football club in case he is doing the same thing to someone else right now.'

He was still squeezing my arm when he'd finished talking. We sat again in silence. I tried to digest the magnitude of what he was telling me. I felt my stomach flip and my hands begin to moisten. I didn't for one minute doubt what Derek had just told me was the truth. I looked at him, crushed, and slumped in his chair. His eyes filled with tears before he used his finger and thumb to grind them away. My mind raced with a thousand disconnected thoughts.

Poor Derek. What a burden to have carried. What evil to have endured as a boy. This monster is still working at Newcastle United. How many other boys has he abused before and after Derek? How close had I come, as a 16-year-old, to being a victim myself? I'd walked straight into the lion's den. What's the next step? We must report it to the police.

I turned to Derek. His hands were failing in their job of stemming the flow from his eyes. His shoulders were heaving as he let go of it all, right there in the middle of the empty pub. Two regulars walked in and waved to me. They looked at Derek and then each other before settling at the bar. They looked again. I tapped Derek's leg.

'Let's have a walk to my house. Let you clear your head. We can have a cup of tea. I might even have some beers in the fridge.'

We strolled the short distance lost in our thoughts. When we got in, he settled for a beer. I spoke to Geraldine in the kitchen and asked her to go and visit a friend for an hour. The look on her face when she'd greeted Derek at the front door suggested she knew all was not well. She left us in the living room of our home in Horsley. Conor was in bed and Owen was still small enough to be asleep in his cot.

Derek sat opposite me. He made me promise again not to tell anyone what he was divulging. He only wanted Ormond out of the football club. With my promise delivered, we spent the night talking and drinking. Or rather Derek spent the night talking. I spent the night listening.

That night I bore witness to the most gut-wrenching testimony I've ever heard from a fellow human being. The sordid detail of the evil depravity a paedophile had inflicted mercilessly on a defenceless child. That child now sat sobbing in my living room as a hollowed-out shell of a man. The Derek I had known was gone. He no longer existed. The new Derek in front of me was still in the midst of his ordeal. Still in the clutches of his tormentor. The man who sat in front of me was utterly changed from the boy I had met in 1981. As the night wore on, and the alcohol began to take its effect, I found out all too well just how much he was changed. I don't know at what point it happened. But at some point in the evening I'd failed to give the right response to a question, or I'd failed to recognise a name Derek had introduced into the conversation. His mood darkened and it darkened very quickly. One minute, we were two old friends trying to make sense of the horrors one of us had experienced, and the next he was a picture of simmering rage.

'You know who I'm talking about and you know what I mean! You know! You fucking know!'

He was sitting upright, staring across the short distance between our chairs and getting very angry with me. I had no idea who or what he was talking about. I decided the best course of action was to pretend I did know what he was talking about after all.

I managed to placate him with an apology for whatever misunderstanding had occurred. I then sat for another uncomfortable hour with him while he glared at me, tapped a beer bottle off my living room wall, and gently boiled. I had two kids upstairs and a menacing, drunken presence sitting right below them. My purgatory was broken by Geraldine's key in the door. His mood lightened when she came into the living room. She offered him a lift home. I discreetly shook my head at her. I convinced him a taxi was on its way. When he'd closed the door behind him, I felt a confusing mixture of emotions. Disgust and anger that this horror had destroyed him. Concern about what could actually be done if he wasn't willing to move forward and tell the police of the crimes committed against him. I was also ashamed of the surge of relief I felt that this menacing ball of anger had finally left my home.

I told Geraldine the bare minimum of what had transpired, and we made our way to bed. I awoke after a restless night's sleep. I lay in bed for a while to rid myself of the grogginess of the beer. I replayed Derek's revelations in my head. I thought about the promises I had made not to divulge our conversation to anyone. I thought long and hard about it. Then I came to the conclusion that I needed to tell someone about the allegations against George Ormond. There was an alleged paedophile working with boys at Newcastle United Football Club. I resolved to break Derek's trust. Some promises were made to be broken.

CHAPTER 27

Newcastle United in 1997 was a club still basking in the glory of the Kevin Keegan 'entertainers' era. Kevin had departed early in the New Year and was replaced by Kenny Dalglish, who went on to lead the team to its second top-two finish in two seasons. These were heady days for the club. It was the team of Shearer, Ferdinand, Ginola, Beardsley and a brilliant supporting cast. But although the team was hitting the heights, behind the scenes our training and medical facilities were bottom of the league. The senior players trained at our rented facility at Maiden Castle in Durham. Our superstar footballers, who'd set the world alight the previous season, only to falter at the final hurdle and finish second to an Eric Cantona-inspired Manchester United, did so in spite of the substandard training facility they worked from every day. The players, now bolstered by the arrival of the world's most expensive footballer, Alan Shearer, trained every day next to often-bewildered Durham University students at their campus sports facility. The indoor facilities were the equivalent of a council-run sports hall. The medical room was comprised of two small offices knocked into one. The players changed in two rented rooms next to the students. The training pitches were of great quality but there simply weren't enough of them to accommodate both the senior players and juniors. So Newcastle United was a club split in two back then. The youth team trained at an entirely different location to the rest of the club and the youth team management office was situated off a long corridor at St James' Park.

When I arrived at training the morning after Derek Bell's shocking revelations, my first task was to find out whether or not George Ormond worked for the club. I had seen him on occasion, in a Newcastle United bench coat, walking around on match days at St James' Park. I was aware that he had done some odd jobs for the youth team management team of John Murray and John Carver, but I had no idea to what extent or in what capacity he was actually employed by the club. If I was going to break Derek Bell's trust, which I'd decided I was going to do, then I needed to know if the alleged paedophile was actually working for the club at the other site. A quick word with my physio colleague and good friend Derek Wright established that Ormond was indeed employed as a masseur/gopher with the youth team. An inquisitive look from my friend ensured he would be the first person to whom I would betray Derek's trust. Derek Wright was unequivocal in his response.

'You have to go to the police with this.'

We were drinking coffee in the upstairs canteen watching an ultra-competitive five-a-side game being played at break-neck speed. Derek was shaking his head and rubbing his face. I shared his reasoning.

'He's told me not to say anything as he's not ready to come forward yet. But I agree that the allegations are so serious that I have to tell the police.'

It was a Thursday morning, and we discussed our options. Our first thoughts were that I should travel into Newcastle, or to Durham, to speak to someone about the information I was in possession of. We resolved that the best course of action was to speak with a senior officer, on Saturday at our next home game, and ask his advice on the next steps to be taken.

On the morning of the game we had breakfast in the players' lounge. I broke Derek Bell's trust again and shared the information and the plan with the kit manager, Ray Thompson. He was both a friend and a confidant. He too was in no doubt that what I was proposing to do was the right course of action. Once the match got underway and the crowd had settled, I asked one of the officers in charge of crowd control if I might have a confidential conversation with him. I told him an allegation of historic sexual abuse had been made by Derek Bell against George Ormond, who was currently working for the youth team. I also told him that Derek had insisted that I tell no one, as he wasn't willing to make a complaint or make his allegations public. The officer listened to me and agreed that I'd done the right thing in divulging the information against the express wishes of Derek, the alleged abuse victim. He asked me to leave the matter with him.

Two weeks later we were back in the same spot at the same time. The frantic early exchanges of the game boomed up the tunnel almost drowning out our conversation. The senior officer explained that he had made some enquiries about Ormond and that he was not on any database. He went on to say that if the person I'd mentioned wanted to come forward with his complaint, then the police would investigate it immediately. If he was not willing to come forward and make an official complaint, then there was nothing the police could do. He suggested that Ormond should be removed from the club.

I was a little taken aback and more than a little disappointed with the advice.

The loud roar of the crowd celebrating a goal ended our conversation. I followed the officer back to our vantage point next to the dugout. We never spoke about George Ormond again.

Two days later I was back at a deserted St James' Park. I hurried past the location of my two conversations with the officer. I made my way along the corridor to the office shared by the youth management team. The cramped office that was overflowing with bibs, balls and cones. John Murray, the Youth Development Officer, and my long-time friend John Carver, the Youth Team Coach, were seated half-hidden in the mess. They listened, in stunned silence, as I relayed Derek Bell's accusations, my subsequent conversations with the senior officer, and his recommendation that George Ormond should be removed from his position at the club. It was a particularly confusing conversation for John Carver, who'd played with Derek, at Montague, under the watchful eye of Ormond. John had remained friends with both men. He was visibly shaken as he spoke in response to my horrific offering.

'I cannot believe it. I cannot believe it. They are mates. They have always been mates. Derek was George's best man. I was drinking in the Black Bull with them both last Sunday night. Why didn't Derek speak to me? I need to speak to Derek. I need to hear it from him. This is unbelievable.'

When he had finished digesting the information and verbalising his disbelief, I reminded him that he couldn't speak with Derek, because for the fourth time in six days, I was breaking his friend's trust. We agreed before I left the room that George Ormond had to be removed from the club.

He was eventually removed from the club, but not before attending a summer youth team tournament in Northern Ireland. In those days, the youth team had no designated physiotherapist, so I was seconded for the trip to the prestigious Milk Cup Tournament in Coleraine. I found myself part of a four-man management team looking after the under-18's, alongside John Murray, John Carver and George Ormond.

To say I was a little uncomfortable that Ormond was on the trip wouldn't come close to what I was feeling. I could barely look at the man. I had a very strong reason to believe he was a monster. Yet here I was working alongside him. We had an initial team debriefing at the hotel. The two Johns were laying the ground rules for the trip. When they'd finished, I asked permission to speak.

'I know you're all not used to having a physio with you and you ordinarily rely on George for massages and sorting out bumps and bruises. I just wanted to say to you all, George included, that all physiotherapy matters are to be referred to me. There is no reason for anyone to be in your rooms other than when you have requested it.'

Apart from telling the world my suspicions, it was the best I could do in the circumstances. The boys headed to their chalets while the staff made our way to our rooms in the main hotel. After emptying my suitcase, I grabbed my first aid kit and headed to the chalets. One of the boys had a wound on his knee that required a clean dressing. I knocked on the door and opened it as I did so. The three boys who were sharing the room were all lying on their beds. The room was already a mess. Clothes and half-opened suitcases already occupied all of the floor space. As I stepped in, I could feel my pulse quicken and my neck hair bristle. There, perched on the end of one of the boy's beds was Ormond. I felt sick. I summoned him outside.

'What are you doing?'

He smiled.

'Relax, Ferra man. I was just seeing if the lad needed his dressing changed. I always change the dressing and do the first aid stuff. I thought I was helping.'

I politely reminded him of the instruction I had just delivered to everyone, including him. He apologised and agreed not to visit the boys' rooms again. I made my way back to my room, hating the fact that he was there and that I was having to police him. A couple of pints into the welcome dinner at the hotel and I began to finally relax. The officials from the various teams were making merry at the inaugural dinner. A few more pints and a hearty meal later, I got up to say my goodnights to John Carver and John Murray, who were next to me. Finally, I said goodnight to Geor... an empty chair!

'Where's George?'

I was up on my feet and on my way as the two Johns answered.

'Probably in the toilet.'

'Maybe at the bar?'

I jogged the short distance to the chalets. The beer swilled in my bloated stomach. I knocked loudly on the door of the same chalet I'd visited earlier. The door opened. Ormond, the man who I believed had abused my friend, the man I had spoken to the police about, the man I had told his coaches about, the man I had found in this room this afternoon, the man who shouldn't be on this trip, was standing in his black-tie dinner suit grinning at me. I'd told him twice only hours before not to visit those rooms. Yet here he was again. I could feel the anger building, my inhibitions lowered by the night's drinking. His smiling face was right in front of me. My teeth were grinding till they hurt. I wanted to crash my head against his nose and feel the satisfaction of it shattering under the force. Then I wanted to kick his tumbling body all over the messy room and drag his rump out of there in full humiliating view of the boys. I took a deep breath and looked over his shoulder.

'Everything OK boys?'

The deep breath hadn't fully done its job. Head-butting his nose was still under consideration. I needed to get him out of there before the boys got to witness the possible end of my career as a physiotherapist at Newcastle United. I took his arm and pulled him out of the room. I walked until we were out of earshot of the chalets.

'What the fuck are you doing back in that room when I told you twice not to go there?'

'Come on, Ferra man. I was just checking they were all alright and didn't need anything.'

I grabbed his arm in the darkness of the hotel car park.

'I'm telling you this for the very last time. Stay out of the boys' rooms for the rest of this trip, or I will...'

'You will what?'

His interruption and the arrogance of his tone shocked me. It sobered me.

I wanted to say, 'I will tell the world that I know you are a paedophile and you abused my friend.' I didn't though, because I didn't know that for certain. I knew nothing for certain. So instead of accusing him of being a paedophile, I threatened him in time honoured drunken tradition.

'I will kick your fucking head in. You arrogant cunt!'

I let go of his arm. He mumbled something as he walked away.

I chased after him and spun him around.

'Are we clear?'

He lowered his head.

'We're clear.'

George Ormond was removed from the club sometime into the new season. I never heard of him again, until 2001, when Derek Bell finally found the courage to tell the police of his ordeal. Under a promise of anonymity, he bravely faced his tormentor in court. In 2002, Ormond was found guilty of abusing Derek and six other boys. He was sentenced to six years in prison. Then in 2016, amid a flurry of allegations from several men who had been abused at various professional clubs, Derek Bell shared his ordeal with the press. It opened the floodgates. Several men came forward to claim that Ormond had abused them when they were boys at Montague Boys' Club and at Newcastle United. When I gave my evidence in 2018, the defence barrister told me that Ormond didn't dispute my account, but he just couldn't remember any of the conversations we'd had. I told her that was alright. My memory was good enough for the both of us.

In July 2018, George Ormond was found guilty of committing 36 counts of sexual abuse, against 18 victims over a 24-year period, between 1973 and 1997. I had indeed walked into the lion's den in 1981. I was lucky. I was not one of his victims. It was clear that I was, after all, dealing with a monster in 1997, when Derek Bell had confided in me and I'd reported his sickening allegations to the police. Ormond was sentenced to 20 years for his crimes. He deserves every minute of it. Derek Bell, and the others, got a life sentence. They don't deserve a second of it.

CHAPTER 28

The Ormond trial, and my ongoing medical issues, made for a miserable summer in 2018. The awards and plaudits for *The Boy on the Shed* continued to provide some much-needed escapism. The book was declared *The Times* Sports Book of the Year. This unexpected accolade was quickly followed by the announcement that it was also *The Sunday Times* Sports Book of the Year. I was surprised and elated by both awards. Winning any kind of award for my writing was way down my list of priorities when I was completing the manuscript. Finding an agent to represent me was the only thing I was thinking of at that time. I wasn't too sure I would be able to do that even. I had no confidence at all that what I had written had enough merit to achieve my first goal. Then when I'd secured Guy Rose as my agent, I was doubtful, in spite of his great confidence, that he would find anyone to publish it. When Hodder and Stoughton had acquired the book, my honest hope was that it would sell enough copies to earn out the advance they'd paid. Not because I was desperate for the money, but because I felt that if the book earned out the advance, then that was a sign it had outperformed Hodder and Stoughton's hopes for it. It was only at that moment that I would regard the book as any kind of success. Now it had exceeded all my expectations.

As time passed, and the reviews continued to be overwhelmingly positive, I allowed myself to relax in the belief that, at the very least, I hadn't written a dreadful book. I started to have faith that *The Boy on the Shed* had been worth writing and deserved its place at the top of the sales charts. I still had no expectations, however, that it might be worth a nomination for any literary awards. Then *The Times* and

The Sunday Times announcements changed all of that. The awards raised my expectations for the book. If it was good enough to achieve such recognition, then what else might be possible for it? I was soon to find out.

Roddy Bloomfield emailed to inform me that the book had made the shortlist for the prestigious *William Hill Sports Book of the Year 2018*. The William Hill award was by far the most coveted sports book award in the world. I remember Nick Hornby's *Fever Pitch* winning it years ago and it led that author into a new life of writing, film scripts and movies. I could only dare to dream of hitting such heights. For now, being one of the six shortlisted titles was enough. The fact that my book had already come out on top in *The Times* and *The Sunday Times* added to my growing sense of anticipation and confidence that it might actually win the *William Hill Sports Book of the Year,* as well. The recognition would be amazing – the £30,000 prize money would be alright, too. I was already guaranteed £3,000 and a leather-bound copy of my book just for making it to the final six. The ceremony was to be held at the British Academy of Film and Television Arts (BAFTA), on Piccadilly in London.

In the weeks and months leading up to the ceremony I put it all out of my mind. Instead, I concentrated on my work at Speedflex, which acted as my main distraction from my low moods and where I was at with my health. We were making such good progress on the work front that the opening of a new Speedflex studio at Bannatyne's Health Club in Belfast threatened to clash with the big day at BAFTA. If I was unable to reconcile the dates then my work at Speedflex had to take priority over an awards ceremony, no matter how much I would like to attend. I'd put far too much work into making Speedflex the success I felt it should be to miss out on anything to do with the progress of our company. But I was also determined to be at BAFTA, for the once-in-a-lifetime chance of seeing my book crowned the Sports Book of the Year. Finally, after a lot of anxious to-ing and fro-ing, I managed to arrange the big launch of our studio for the day before the awards ceremony in London. I asked Alan Shearer to travel with us to Belfast to add some stardust to the launch. I'd then have a few celebratory drinks and get to bed early. I would be up and on my way to Heathrow long before the rest of our party were shaking off their hangovers over a cooked breakfast at the hotel.

The week before the award ceremony the book picked up another literary prize. It was announced as *The Daily Telegraph* Football Book of the Year, for 2018. A review in *The Sunday Times* of all the William Hill contenders declared *The Boy on the Shed* as the favourite to win. A doctor's appointment letter arrived on the morning of my two-day trip to Belfast and London. It was confirmation of my upcoming consultation to discuss the merits of a bionic penis. Not a great date for anyone's diary, unless you're The Six Million Dollar Man, I suppose. Every time I received these hospital letters they dampened my spirits. They were a constant reminder of my reality. I wasn't exactly looking forward to what was guaranteed to be another embarrassing conversation about the sorry state of my downstairs department. I resolved not to let it spoil what promised to be a brilliant two days for me. I scanned it, put the date in my diary and threw the letter on the kitchen windowsill as I made my way out the door.

As I set out for Belfast and then London nothing was going to quell my excitement at what was to come for me. We flew to Dublin, and then bussed up to Belfast. It was the only way we could get Alan there on the night in question. Any other day, and any other way, and I wouldn't have been able to get to London on time. Geraldine had been invited to the William Hill awards ceremony, too. She was as excited as me to go and experience something that may never happen in our lives again. Then she got a call to say her school was being visited by Ofsted on the day of the ceremony. She had been reluctant to take a day off anyway, but the Ofsted call guaranteed my wife would not be with me in London after all. She'd always behaved like the entire school system would collapse if she missed a day's work. Don't let anyone ever tell you teachers are not dedicated. Much to my frustration, she'd never take a day off for any reason. I could see now that not even an invitation to a swanky awards ceremony at BAFTA could change that. Conor agreed to be my plus-one in her absence. He'd travel from Newcastle and meet Roddy, Karen and Guy at midday for the drinks and canapés that preceded the big announcement at 2 p.m. My 8 a.m. flight would unfortunately mean that I would be there far too early. I would have to occupy myself in London for a little while before making my way to the venue.

The launch of the Speedflex studio went very smoothly. Alan was his usual accommodating self. He trained in the studio with members of the Bannatyne's Health Club, where our brand-new studio now dominated the entrance to the impressive building. He gave his time generously after the session, to anyone who approached him. He spoke with the local press about his ongoing commitment to the adventure we were on with our exciting concept. Then afterwards we headed into Belfast for a night out with the Bannatyne's team. I loved being in Belfast and I loved the fact that our latest and most impressive studio to date was in my home country. All those years ago, when I'd left as a timid 16-year-old determined to make my way in professional football, I couldn't have envisaged returning one day as the CEO of such an exciting young company. Not only that, I was returning with one of the country's most successful businessmen, Graham Wylie, as my partner and funder. I was also coming home with England's greatest-ever centre forward as a fellow director, but more importantly as my very good friend.

I really enjoyed my night out in Belfast, a city I don't know very well. It was only eight miles from my hometown of Lisburn, but I rarely visited it during The Troubles in the late 1970s and I was gone by 1981. I never got to grow up in this great city of music and culture, and had only socialised in it as an adult on one or two occasions when I had been home to visit family in Lisburn. I had done my growing up in another great city, many miles away in England. I had grown to love my adopted city of Newcastle, with its beautiful architecture, friendly people, passion for football and its own unique culture. But as I sat in the cosy bar in Belfast, with the Guinness flowing and my friends laughing, I felt a pang of regret for the life I never got to live there. I was a stranger in my own land. The streets and pubs that my parents grew up in were alien to me. I would never share their experience. I was no longer part of the tribe. My children were Geordies. The streets and pubs they frequented were the same ones I had visited as a young man at their age.

After snapping out of my daydream, I went on to drink one or two too many pints. I knew I'd done so as soon as I got up from the glass strewn table. Not because my head was spinning or I had to be carried home. I knew I'd drunk too much because of the first drops that leaked into the place where my pad should have been. *My pad!* I'd forgotten to wear my bloody pad. In the previous few weeks I'd taken to not wearing my pads. Mostly I'd stayed dry, apart from an embarrassing leakage at the checkout in Morrisons when I'd dribbled through my jeans as I bent over to get some stubborn biscuits that had jammed in the trolley. I covered myself with my shopping as I leaked down my leg all the way to the sanctuary of my car. The only time I made sure I wore one was if I was going on a night out. I was still scarred by my Killarney experience, where I'd pissed like a fountain all the way back to the hotel from the pub. I never wanted to repeat that performance but here I was in the pub in Belfast, about to do the same thing again. Maybe it was Ireland that brought the worst out in me?

As I took my first step towards the door and the taxi home, I felt the trickle become a pour. I pretended to tie my laces so the others would move in front of me and I followed them to the waiting car. I cursed my stupidity. I hadn't so much forgotten to wear my pad this time as made a conscious decision not to do so. My logic, in the hotel room before going to the launch, was that if I didn't wear a pad, then I wouldn't drink too much alcohol. If I didn't drink too much alcohol, then I would be up bright and early to head to London. A good plan sabotaged by Arthur Guinness.

It was with great relief that I finally made it back to my room. The bemused look on Alan's face when I'd declined his offer of a nightcap in the hotel bar was matched by all of the others who accepted his invitation. I couldn't accept. My jeans were drenched.

'Goodnight, you miserable bastard. Hope your book wins tomorrow. It deserves to.'

That was my disappointed friend's parting shot as I scurried off to the lift. I held my jacket in front of me to cover the ever-growing wet patch on my jeans. I showered and put a pad on for bed. The embarrassment of potentially leaking over hotel sheets guaranteed I always wore my pads at night. I set my alarm for 6 a.m. and allowed myself to dream of glory the following day. It promised to be one of the most memorable of my life. People from my background don't usually win prestigious literary prizes. I tossed and turned before finally falling asleep and awoke exhausted, but very excited about the day that lay ahead of me. I made the short trip from hotel to airport.

'Are you nervous?'

'Yes please.'

'What?'

'Do you want beans?'

'A little bit maybe.'

'What?'

'Yes please?'

'Are you alright?'

'No sausage thanks.'

'Do you want me to call back?'

'Tea please.'

'Paul?'

'Thank you.'

'Paul, I'll call back.'

'Don't hang up! Sorry Geraldine. I shouldn't have answered. I was in the queue at the airport restaurant. My flight gets called soon and I didn't want to miss you before you go off to work. How are you?'

'I'm OK. I didn't sleep very well with nerves. When you didn't call, I presumed you'd drunk too much and was worried you'd sleep in.'

I spoke between mouthfuls.

'You were right on the first count. I drank so much I wet myself.'

'You didn't? Were you wearing your pad?'

'That would have been far too sensible.'

'Oh shit. Did anybody notice?'

'Me and my jeans did.'

'You know what I mean.'

'You mean, did I embarrass myself? No. I didn't embarrass myself.'

She could sense my angst.

'Listen. I know it's shit and I know it hurts you, but as long as you're healthy and the cancer is gone I don't care if you piss yourself every day. Don't let it spoil today for you. It's a bloody amazing achievement to be shortlisted, never mind win the thing. Promise me you'll enjoy every minute of it. It doesn't happen every day you know. Besides, every other woman you walk past today has been in the same boat as you. If they've had a child, then they may well have had to wear a pad at some stage, believe me.'

She was right but I hated having the conversation we were having. I didn't want my wife to be asking me if I had worn my pad, or if anyone had noticed my leakage. I didn't want to be having those discussions with her, or anybody, but especially not her. This was the girl I'd grown up with, the girl I got dressed up for, the woman I'd married, my soulmate. The last thing I'd ever envisaged would be that she would become my confidant in matters of incontinence, erectile dysfunction, penile shrinkage, and the mental turmoil that goes with that lot. I still wanted to be the boy who'd made her heart skip a beat as she passed me in the street; the boy she longed for on those long lonely nights after I'd left for England; the boy she'd left Ireland for to be with. I wanted to be the man she'd married, had kids with and relied on to help her build a life for our family. I wanted us to grow old together, to have adventures. To see the world side by side after the kids had upped and left. And yes, I wanted us to still be intimate with each other. We *were* still intimate with each other. Just not in the way we used to be. Secretly confiding to the love of your life that you've wet yourself again is not the sort of intimacy I was hoping for. Nor was it what she would have dreamed of.

She wished me well for the exciting day ahead. She told me she loved me and hung up. I missed the tannoy announcement that my flight was ready for boarding. I tidied my half-eaten breakfast away and got ready to head for departures. I felt a rush of excitement for what was to come. I glanced at the screen above me. I checked again to make sure the information displayed was correct. It read:

Air Lingus, flight 331, to London Heathrow. CANCELLED.

Not ready for boarding. Not delayed. CANCELLED.

FUCKING CANCELLED.

CHAPTER 29

George Best Airport, in Belfast, is so small that you can sprint from the restaurant to the back of the Aer Lingus cancelled flight queue in less than 10 seconds. I sprinted so fast that I only stopped when I ran into the back of a large American woman. She interrupted her loud whining to her equally large husband to give me a look that said one step further and I'll eat you too. I raised my hands.

'I'm so sorry – didn't see you.'

She looked herself up and down.

'Really, buddy?'

I stuttered.

'Well. I did see you. Obviously, I saw you. I mean – not obviously. What I meant to say was I was in such a rush that I just couldn't stop.'

She smiled.

'Relax, buddy. I'm just messing with ya. Bad news about the flight. Looks like another day in Belfast for us. What about you? Anything important happening in London?'

I digested the information. Another day in Belfast. I was going to miss it, my big day at BAFTA, probably my only day at BAFTA. My smiling American was staring at me, waiting for my reply. I shook my head.

'No, nothing important in London. Another day in Belfast for me, too.'

She turned to nag her husband. I waited impatiently for the queue to disappear until it was my turn to speak to the flustered young girl behind the counter. By the time I got to her she was in a particularly unhelpful mood.

'The flight is cancelled due to fog in London. The British Airways flight that departed five minutes ago was operating under British Airways policy. Aer Lingus policy is to cancel. I know it is the same fog in London, but our policy is to cancel. There is another flight at 3.20 p.m. but it is likely to be full. Sorry for the inconvenience. Collect your bag from our desk to the left. Next?'

I resisted the urge to lecture her on manners and customer service and instead shuffled off to join the other queue to retrieve my bag. I dragged it across to the nearest empty chair. I fell into it and looked for Karen's number to let her know I wouldn't be joining her in London today. An important-looking, perfectly coiffured gentleman was occupying the seat next to me. He was all teeth and tan. He talked confidently and calmly into his phone.

'Hi, Jen. Aer Lingus flight to Heathrow has been cancelled. Can you contact my 11.30 a.m. appointment at the Mandarin Oriental and let them know I'll likely be there at 1.30 p.m. instead?'

1.30? Today? Private jet maybe?

'I'm heading to the international airport now. Book me on the next flight out of there this morning.'

I felt my heart pumping. *Aldergrove!* Why hadn't I thought of that? There must be flights out of there to London this morning. All was not lost. Why didn't the unhelpful girl behind the desk tell me that? Oh yes, probably because she was unhelpful. I scrambled through my phone. I called Sinead, our office manager, at Speedflex. She would sort it. She was brilliant at sorting things. She was used to sorting things for me because I was useless at sorting things. Not everything. Just everything to do with the modern world of technology we now live in. Her phone rang and rang and rang again. *Fuck!* I rang Vikki. Vikki was our Speedflex marketing manager. She was back at the hotel, most probably sleeping. She was also very good at this modern world thing. She was also well used to dealing with me in a flap. It had been five years since she'd sat on the end of my desk, as a 23-year-old, and talked calmly to me after I'd told her I was having chest pains, which I now suspect was a heart attack, just two days before I had the one that nearly killed me. Vikki was good in a crisis. She answered on the first ring.

'Hello. What? Shit! What are you going to do?'

As she was talking, Sinead's number flashed up on my phone. I now had two capable helpers on the case.

'Why don't you jump in a taxi and head to the international airport? Me and Sinead will try and work something out so that you can still get to the awards ceremony for 12.'

I thanked her and made my way to the taxi rank. *No taxis.* I called the number from the Freephone. I waited for five minutes that seemed like 50. I didn't say a word to the driver on the whole 30-minute ride. My stomach was churning, and I could feel a trickle of sweat run down my forehead. I stared at my phone waiting for the call from Sinead or Vikki. Five minutes from the terminal, it finally came. It was Sinead.

'Good news. There are two flights out of the international. One at 10 a.m., with easyJet, to Gatwick. The other at 10.15 a.m., with British Airways, to Heathrow. I think both will get you into London in time for the awards at 12.'

I looked at my watch. It was 9.15. I looked up and the airport was visible in the distance.

'Have I time to book onto the easyJet one?'

'You'll be cutting it fine. I can't buy a ticket online. You'll have to go to easyJet customer services and buy one in the airport.'

I can't remember if I thanked her and don't know how much money I threw into the front of the taxi as he pulled up outside the airport. It must have been enough though as he didn't follow me into the terminal. I headed towards the departure desk before remembering that I needed to go to customer services. I'm not good in a flap! There was no one on the desk when I got to it. I could hear voices coming from the brightly-lit booth behind it.

'Hello… hello… excuse me… excuse me… hello!'

A smartly dressed girl popped out of the booth. I told her of my urgent need to get to London this morning. I also told her I would marry her if she could sort it. Then I remembered that I was now a middle-aged man breathing heavily and sweating – I definitely sounded a bit creepy. I was going for funny – but I think I landed on creepy. I retracted the last statement and apologised. She smiled, unoffended, and got to work.

'It will cost you £96 for the ticket, which I will issue here. If you only have hand luggage, just go straight to departures as the flight will be boarding shortly.'

I ran up the escalator that led to the notoriously slow security check area at Belfast. There were times in the recent past when I'd queued there for nearly an hour. Even 20 minutes would be too much today. I zig-zagged my way around the endless barriers and entered the security checking area. I looked up to assess the length of the queue. There was no one there. Not one passenger. Just another four columns of barriers to navigate. I slapped my bag, boots, wallet and phone in the basket and met them on the other side of the scanner. I breathed a deep sigh as I made my way into the terminal. I'd made it!

Thanks to Vikki, Sinead, the taxi driver, and the young girl, who'd briefly received a marriage proposal from a fat 50-something man, I was going to the ball after all. I strolled through the gift shop and headed for Starbucks. I scanned the departure board. I found my flight. *Call for departure is 8 minutes.* Not only had I made it, but I even had time for a well-earned coffee. I brought my coffee out of Starbucks, sat on a bench and exhaled. What a bloody palaver. I brought the hot liquid to my lips and looked for my flight on the board. It was flashing red. Red is never good. It wasn't.

Flight delayed. Expected departure time 10.30 a.m. A voice came over the tannoy.

'Would all passengers travelling to London Heathrow, on flight BA345, please make their way to gate 18. This flight is now ready for boarding.'

I pointed aimlessly at the screen and laughed. I only stopped laughing when I sensed the elderly couple sitting next to me moving away from me. The British Airways flight, scheduled after mine, was now departing before mine. The British Airways flight this morning had departed as scheduled. Mine was cancelled. What was it with British Airways? Did its planes have better fog lights?

I sipped my coffee and worked out my times. If my flight departed at 10.30 a.m. I would be cutting it fine but might still make the presentation at 2 p.m. I resisted the urge to call my editor and publicist to let them know their author was stuck in Belfast because Aer Lingus and easyJet aren't as fond of fog as British Airways. It was a good decision as my flight was called just as I finished my coffee. I was finally on my way to London.

I boarded the plane, squeezed into my window seat, and breathed a huge sigh of relief as I fastened my seatbelt ready for take-off. With a fair wind, I still had a chance of making the ceremony. I was so desperate to be there, not only to hopefully win the award, but just to be part of a literary event. I allowed myself to envisage strolling on to the stage, rapturous applause ringing in my ears.

When I snapped out of my imaginary acceptance speech, I was surprised to see we were still on the tarmac. I checked the time on my phone. It had been 15 minutes since the doors had closed and the pilot had instructed us to watch and listen closely to the flight attendant. It didn't take me long to fathom that if we didn't take off very soon, I had little or no chance of making the start of the presentation. In fact, even if we took off that very minute then I probably still had little chance. I suddenly felt very hot. I reached up and twiddled with the air conditioner. It didn't respond. I checked my phone again. Then the captain interrupted my latest flap.

'Ladies and gentlemen: very sorry for the delay. We have been in communication with Gatwick trying to sort out a slot. They have finally given us one and I have good news and bad news. We can still make our way to London this morning, but I'm afraid you will have to sit back and relax for a little while. It will be 45 minutes from now until we take off.'

I could barely hear the rest of his instruction over the murmuring buzz in the cabin and the thumping of my heart which was pounding in my ears.

'I will update you with any progress. Meanwhile, sit back, relax and enjoy your flight when we eventually make our way to Gatwick.'

I sunk into my chair and cursed the world. I cursed the fact that I'd travelled to Ireland the day before the awards, I cursed

Aer Lingus. I cursed myself for not booking British Airways with its better pilots and superior fog lights. I cursed easyJet and its useless air conditioning, and I cursed William Hill and its stupid awards ceremony, which had allowed me to dream of what would undoubtedly be one of the best days of my life. When I'd stopped cursing, I checked my times again. I'd definitely missed the ceremony – that much was clear. Conor would be there for it, alongside Guy, Roddy and Karen. But I could still make the announcement of the winner and would be there for the celebrations to follow. That was still something to look forward to.

I called Karen and updated her on the ridiculous turn of events that meant her author wasn't going to make the ceremony, but still had a chance of getting there for the announcement at 2 p.m. She said she would organise a car to collect me from Victoria Station. I settled down to sweat my way through the next 40 minutes. I dozed off and was awoken by the pilot's voice.

'Ladies and gentlemen, the situation with the fog in London is a movable feast. As such, we will be disembarking the aircraft in five minutes. Thank you.'

I felt my heart in my ears again. *Disembarking? Jesus Christ. Could this day get any worse?* I felt like head-butting the seat in front of me. I settled for clenching every clenchable part of me. I added some silent screaming. The plane was noisy with chatter and hurried phone calls. I called Karen. I was in the middle of telling her that I was now getting off my plane and wouldn't be meeting her in London after all, when the pilot spoke again and forced me to hang up.

'Sorry, ladies and gentlemen. The cabin crew have informed me that I may have caused a little confusion with my terminology. When I said disembarking, I meant to say that the fog in London has cleared, and we have been given an earlier slot. We will be making our way to the westerly runway in approximately five minutes time. We hope to have you on the ground in the capital at approximately 1.20 p.m.'

My relief that we were finally taking off quickly fizzled when I worked out that there was simply no way I could make it from the airport to the awards for 2 p.m. I spoke to the girl in the middle seat next to me. I just needed to share my pain and frustration with somebody. I'd missed my big day and I would most probably never have another. The well-dressed, middle-aged businessman in the aisle seat then leaned forward.

'Sorry. I couldn't help overhearing your conversation. It would be a real shame for you to miss out on something like that. I live in London through the week and travel this route all the time. If you would like, I could try and get you to the awards for 2 p.m.?'

'Really? Do you think it is still possible?'

He raised his eyebrow.

'It'll be tight. Can you run?'

'I can run.'

'Then let's get you there.'

I calmed my racing pulse and called Karen to tell her the plan. I would do my best to meet her at 2 p.m. for the announcement. I willed the plane into the air and coaxed it all the way to London. All was not lost. It really is the hope that kills you.

CHAPTER 30

His name was Robert, and he was as good as his word. As soon as the plane's wheels touched the tarmac, we were ready and primed for the fasten seatbelts signs to disappear. They had barely gone off before we were up and away, much to the obvious annoyance of some of the other passengers. We skipped past 10 rows of heads before any of them were out of their seats. The doors opened and we were off. He led and I followed close behind. There was a long incline from the plane to the main terminal. That ramp ensured I was in no position to speak to Robert when he occasionally glanced back to make sure I was still following. Instead, I just smiled and gulped the stale air. We took left turns, right turns, ascended and descended escalators, and eventually made our way to the doors that led us to the Gatwick Express train. They were just closing as we jumped through them and onto the packed train.

Rivers of sweat were pouring down my forehead and more were making their way down my back. I was breathing heavily and trying to hide that fact from the two middle-aged women I was pressed against. I glanced at one who was staring intensely at me. Her glare made me sweat more and I flared my nostrils in an attempt to calm my breathing. My armpits were soaked and I looked with dread to see if the evidence had made its way on to my new jacket bought especially for today. I wished I hadn't. Two ever expanding semi-circles of wetness, were making their way to the middle of my jacket. If my jacket had been buttoned the circles would have met there. I could feel cold air on my belly. I looked down to see my new shirt flapping open, exposing my all-too-round stomach. The five bullet holes from my prostate surgery were now exposed to the world. No wonder the woman was staring at me. I'd have stared at me too if I wasn't me. I was in the middle of tucking my shirt in with one hand, while holding my suitcase between my knees, and leaning my other arm against the door (I didn't want to raise it because of the sweat patch), when the train rocked to the left. I lost my balance and only regained it again by placing both hands on the shoulders of the staring lady. Thank God she wasn't taller. If she had been then I'd have been in a very awkward situation. I winced, apologised and removed my hands all at the same time. I waited for her to berate me. She lowered her head, opened her handbag and handed me a bottle of water and a packet of handkerchiefs.

'I'm glad I'm not having your day. You look like you need the water.'

I thanked her for her kindness and apologised for the sweat and the near grope. I chatted to her and her friend for the rest of the trip. As we pulled into Victoria Station, they both promised to buy my book, and wished me well.

As the doors opened, I searched for Robert. He was already on the platform. I caught his eye, and the weaving, sweating, slipping and sliding middle-aged duo were off again. We were through the barriers, down the escalator and onto the underground in the blink of an eye. I dabbed the sweat from my forehead and tucked my misbehaving shirt in again. I vowed to get a better fitting shirt, or a smaller belly, before my next sprinting session through London. Robert looked at his watch. It was 1.45 p.m. There were three stops left to our destination. It was two stops too many for us to possibly get there in time.

'We are not going to make it, are we Robert?'

He shook his head. I thanked him for the amazing efforts he'd made on behalf of a total stranger. He'd interrupted his entire day to try to do something genuinely selfless for someone he'd never met and probably never would again. I was still thanking him when we pulled into the next station. The doors opened. With no warning, he grabbed my collar and pulled me off the train. He started running again. I stood still. He turned around to face me.

'Come on Paul. I think we will get there quicker if we grab a taxi outside here. You are only a couple of minutes away.'

I slipped and slid through the crowded platform. I scaled the escalator two stops at a time and jumped in the taxi. It was 1.50 p.m. I had 10 minutes before the big announcement. The taxi weaved its way through static traffic. I started to feel like I might actually get there for the big announcement. Then suddenly the taxi ground to a halt. Robert spoke with the driver and pushed my head against the window.

'Up there on the right. Can you see it? There's the entrance to BAFTA!'

I couldn't see it at first. I couldn't see it because I was looking for some huge building all lit up with bright lights. I think I must have watched too many *Sunday Nights at the London Palladium* when I was younger. I was expecting a grand theatre. I'd only just picked out the door about 50 yards away when Robert was pushing me out of the taxi and into the traffic. I checked the time – 1.58 p.m. I started to run again on what were now very weary legs. I wasn't going to make it for 2. Then I remembered I hadn't even thanked him. I hadn't thanked him for the kindness he'd shown to me as a total stranger. I turned but Robert and his taxi had already left the busy road and were disappearing up a side street. I ran all the way along Piccadilly Street until I was standing outside the door of number 194–195. *The closed door!* I tried the handle. *The locked door!* I looked at my phone to check the time. It was 2.02. I'd missed it! All that stress, all that effort and I had missed a moment I would never have again. The moment when my book, *The Boy on the Shed,* which I had poured my heart and soul into, was crowned the William Hill Sports Book of the Year, 2018. They were probably all toasting my success behind the locked door I was now leaning my head against. I took my frustration out on it and thumped it as hard as I could. Then I winced at the shooting pain in my wrist. I was looking up and down the busy street, wondering what to do, or where to go next, when the door opened. I spoke to the bemused man in front of me.

214

'My name is Paul Ferris. My book is on the shortlist for the award today. I've missed it I know. Could you show me the way to the theatre please?'

He looked at his folder, found my name, and ushered me into the hallway.

'It's on the third floor. There's a lift, but you might be quicker taking the stairs.'

I was already heaving my suitcase up the first flight. They were steep. I was exhausted, but I climbed them as fast as my wobbly legs and tight chest would let me. In no time, I was standing in front of another closed door. I checked the time – 2.10 p.m. I'd missed the big moment by 10 minutes. I could hear talking and loud laughter from inside. I prised the theatre door open. I adjusted my eyes to the darkness in front of me, and then peered into the bright lights of the stage below. TV presenter John Inverdale, the compere, was engaged in an animated and a celebratory conversation with the winning author. My heart dropped into my shoes. As I stared from the shadow at the back of the small theatre, I couldn't help but be crushed by the disappointment of it all.

'You must be Paul?'

A whispering girl with a clipboard rescued me from my misery.

'Yes. I'm Paul.'

John was finishing up with the interview.

'Ladies and gentlemen. Put your hands together once more for Ben Ryan, and his brilliant book, *Sevens Heaven.*'

They shook hands and the applause was loud and lengthy. I pointed to the stage.

'I see I've just missed it then. Seeing the winner crowned.'

She squinted at her watch and then looked at the stage.

'Oh no. We're running about 15 minutes late. You've arrived just in time. That's the last of the on-stage interviews with all the authors. You've missed your slot, but your editor spoke very well on your behalf. Come and I will show you to your seat.'

My heart jumped back to its rightful place. I could feel sweat forming on my forehead for the umpteenth time that day. But this sweat was different. It wasn't fat-middle-aged-man-tearing-across-London sweat. No. This was very different. This was an *I made it* sweat.

I had actually bloody made it! More than that, I had made it just at the perfect time. I had made it for the big reveal. My pulse rate doubled and my breathing joined it, as she guided me into my seat. I shook hands with Guy, Karen and Roddy as I slipped in beside them. I leaned forward and squeezed Conor's shoulders. I was glad he'd made the effort to be there for this occasion. I would have hated to be there with no family to share it with me. I was still squeezing his shoulders when John Inverdale approached the front of the stage. As he started to speak Conor lifted his hand and rested it on mine.

'Ladies and gentlemen, we have reached the stage in the proceedings where it is my great pleasure and honour to be able to announce the winner of the William Hill Sports Book of the Year for 2018.'

I felt like my heart was going to leap out of my throat. My whole head buzzed with nervous excitement.

'All of the judges agree that the standard has been incredibly high this year, and that it was almost impossible to separate the contenders. It was so difficult in fact, that for the first year in its history, the award will go to not just one book, but two books. The two authors will share the £30,000 prize money and the honour of being recognised as the winner of this year's award.'

I squeezed hard on Conor's shoulders. He squeezed hard on my hand. *The Boy on the Shed*, had won every other award. Several times already it had beaten all of the others on the shortlist. Now, there were to be two winners instead of one. One of them was guaranteed to be *The Boy on the Shed*. My planes, trains and automobiles adventure had all been worth it. In fact, it had made the day even more special. John Inverdale interrupted my racing mind.

'Rather than announce the winners, I will just count down from three to one and as if by magic the two winners will flash up on the screen behind me.'

I didn't need to see it on the screen. I didn't need the count down. I *knew* I had won. I *knew* that all of the running about and panicking had led me right to this special moment. I watched the screen to see who the other worthy winner was.

'3... 2... 1'

The screen suddenly lit up. I looked for the familiar cover of my book. I saw the unfamiliar covers of two other books – *A Boy in the Water* and *The Lost Soul of Eamonn Magee*. *The Boy on the Shed* was nowhere to be seen. Instead, its dejected author was shaking hands with his agent, editor and publicist, who were all offering their commiserations.

Talk about a damp squib. It was like a post-prostatectomy orgasm. All of that effort, stress, sweat and anticipation had helped turn the event into the biggest anti-climax of my life. I may as well have stayed in Belfast when the first flight had been cancelled. Now, I faced another trek across London and a three-hour train journey home. It got worse. No sooner had we left the theatre when one of the officials asked me to follow her into another room. There was a camera and a reporter there. They asked if I would hold my book up and answer some questions, as if the award hadn't been announced yet. It was for the highlights reel. I did my duty.

'So Paul, what would it mean to you to win this year's award?'

'It would be the biggest achievement of my entire life. I...'

I was interrupted by a scrum of people passing by me. In the middle of it were the two winning authors. They were smiling and shaking hands. I continued with my explanation of how this promised to be the biggest day of my life. When I had finished speaking, I entered the room where the two winning authors were. I introduced myself, congratulated them both and disappeared into the crowd.

I found my group drinking wine downstairs. A smiling girl gave me a cheque for £3,000 for being a runner-up. She also gave me a £1,000 voucher for a free bet of my choice to be used within 12 months. I said my goodbyes and left with Conor to make our way home. We boarded the train at King's Cross and traipsed through the first-class cabin towards standard class. We walked through two overcrowded cabins before finding seats three rows away from each other. I sat down next to a drunk man who was sucking the life out of a can of Stella Artois. I looked at my cheque, my voucher, and the third part of my prize, a leather-bound copy of my book. I got up, tapped Conor on the shoulder and we made our way to an empty table in first class. As the man with the trolley poured our first half-pints of warm Sauvignon Blanc, I looked at my prizes again. Today wasn't a day to be disappointed. Today was a day to celebrate. For the first time in my life, I'd just won money for my writing. Not as much money as I'd been hoping for, but it was still a prize. A considerable one at that. I didn't know it then but 11 months later the voucher would win me another £6,000. Thank you, Harry Kane!

We drank whatever wine we were given and were a sorry sight when Geraldine picked us up from the station. I crawled into bed and checked my diary. If today had been a strange one, then my next special event promised to be a very surreal one. I had an appointment to see a man about a bionic penis.

CHAPTER 31

The urology waiting area at the Freeman Hospital had become an all-too-familiar place. I sat in the large atrium for what seemed like the hundredth time. I'd first visited it five years earlier when I'd been experiencing some pain from my kidney stone. It was in one of the consultation rooms here that a urologist had stuck his unsolicited finger up my bum. He'd informed me that I had an enlarged prostate, which was quite normal for a man of my age and nothing to worry about. It was in another room off here two years ago that a different urologist told me I had a significant prostate cancer, and that it was definitely something to worry about.

After the failure of the pills and the debacle of the penis pump, I was here to find out a little more about my last resort: having a penile implant inserted. It wasn't a conversation I'd ever imagined having in my life. It wasn't one I was particularly relishing having either. The hour-long wait in the crowded atrium did nothing to ease my anxiety.

'Mr Paul Ferris.'

The stern-looking nurse disturbed me from a light nap. The dribble on my chin had me looking around to see if anyone had been watching the show. The lack of eye contact from the couple opposite gave me my answer. I jumped to attention and smiled nervously at her. Her expression remained the same. She turned and I followed her along the familiar narrow corridor. She stopped at a desk next to three other nurses. They wore a mixture of brown and blue uniforms. She pointed to the open door opposite them.

'Just through there, Mr Ferris.'

I smiled again, thanked her, shuffled past her and her colleagues, and slipped through the door. I was met by the doctor. He shared her facial expression. Not unpleasant, just business-like. He ushered me to the chair just inside the door. It sat at the side of his small desk. On it were several pieces of apparatus. One looked like Concorde standing proudly on a narrow stand. Another, lying beside it, resembled a pencil rolled up in string. And there was a third bit of kit that looked like a pen with a pump attached. I stared at them. I heard a commotion behind me and my eyes followed it. Through the open door I could see the nurses laughing at the latest one-liner one of them had delivered. I felt my cheeks flush. The doctor was unperturbed and started to speak. I tried to listen but I couldn't concentrate on his words. He was asking me a question about orgasms. He asked another about masturbation. He followed that up with another about masturbation, orgasms and erectile dysfunction. The nurses outside the open door laughed again. Not at me. Not at the questions I was being asked. Not at the array of prostheses displayed in full view of them. They were just four friends taking a moment to have a catch-up. Only their catch-up just happened to be right outside the open door of a room where I was engaging in my most embarrassing doctor's appointment since my 'Jack the Diddy Nipper' one.

I looked at the doctor sitting opposite me happily discussing my very sensitive issues in the trouser department. He was oblivious to the open door behind me. I had an overwhelming urge to scream at him. To tell him not to be so uncaring; to close the door on my embarrassment, as a fellow human being. Could he not have some level of understanding about what it feels like to be a man sitting in his office with fake penises strewn across the table? Could he not have some awareness of what it feels like to be talking about dry wanking without an erection, while four young women stood just a few feet away from me were peering through an open door? I can't think of a time when I have felt more humiliated, more insignificant or small. I should have said something. I didn't. Instead, I stared at the open door. He followed my eyes, reached across me and pushed it closed. When he had my attention, he ran through the questions again. When he was satisfied with my answers, he asked me to lie on the bed behind him and slip my jeans and underwear down to my thighs. He washed his hands. He pulled my foreskin back and pinched the top of my penis between his fingers and thumb. He then pulled it straight into the air, stretching it as far as it would go.

'That's the length your penis will be with the implant. The gland here at the top will stay soft with any erection you have in the future.'

It was obviously a line that he had delivered many times to disappointed patients like the one whose penis he was still stretching. I asked a pointless question.

'Is there any chance it can just be the same as it was before?'

He let go of my stretched penis and shook his head.

'I'm afraid not. You have some shrinkage after surgery, which is very common. We can give you an erection again, but we are working with what you have left after surgery. You are two years post-surgery so you shouldn't expect any changes now.'

I pulled my jeans up and made my way to the chair. We had a lengthy discussion about the options open to me, which both you and I will be familiar with by now. I still really didn't fancy the 'rods' option at all. If I was going to go for the reservoir option, then it would most definitely be, *let's scrape all the erectile tissue from your shaft, stick a pouch of liquid in your abdomen and a put a pump in your ballbag.* I asked a few more questions around length (or lack of it), and what an erection looks like when the top of your penis remains soft. His answers didn't have me jumping off the chair ready for yet more surgery. He asked if I had considered injection therapy as an option. I had contemplated it but had dismissed it. I just hadn't fancied the idea of having to stick a needle in the base of my penis every time I wanted to use it. It really hadn't appealed to me that much until now. After weighing up the pros and cons of the implants I got cold feet and agreed to try the injection therapy. It suddenly sounded like it might be the answer after all. I shook the consultant's freshly washed hand and he agreed to see me again after I had tried the injections. He was very thorough and very professional. He was genuinely concerned with finding a solution that worked for me.

I closed his door behind me. I left the hospital a little despondent about the potential of the penile implant, but I was, however, filled with renewed hope that the injection therapy might just work. It was nothing to be frightened of. It was, after all, just a small prick in a small prick.

Christmas 2018 was fast approaching, and I headed from the hospital straight to the madness of the Metrocentre in Gateshead. It was packed with last-minute shoppers and panic buyers like me. I needed a present for Geraldine's mum and dad. Every year played out in the same way. We would be full of grand ideas of getting them something really thoughtful and every year we would give up and order them a hamper from the internet. After two hours of bumping shoulders with half of the north east of England, I gave up. I was due to be in Belfast for work in two days' time. I would buy them something special when I was there and drop into them on my way back to the airport. Two days later I was opening the back door of their home in Lisburn while balancing their thoughtful present on my knee as I did so. The thoughtful present? Oh – a hamper bought from a shop in Bow Street. At least it wasn't off the internet this year.

Mary greeted me in the kitchen. She was in her late 70s but as sprightly as someone 10 years younger. We hugged and I made my way into the familiar living room to see Leo. I found him in his favourite chair, sitting with his back to me. He didn't get up to greet me with his customary hug. As I moved around his chair it didn't take me long to ascertain why. The Leo that I had known for 40 years was no longer there. Instead, there was an old shell. Physically he was unrecognisable. Years of heart failure and recent weight loss had rendered him a bag of bones, unable to stand. An oxygen tank that buzzed by the side of him and fed into his nose was accompanied by a walking frame that rested in front of him. His losing battle with dementia meant our conversation made no sense to either of us. I felt my eyes fill as he forced himself to rise from his chair as I was leaving. I leaned over him and hugged his bones. He whispered, 'Great to see you son.' I was out of the house and into the car before the first tear hit my cheek. I flew home and told Geraldine she needed to go home soon if she ever wanted to see her dad again. We lay in bed and made plans to do just that for New Year. We'd spend Christmas Day with our boys, celebrate Isla's second birthday on the 27th and then fly to Ireland sometime before New Year.

All went to plan. Christmas was great, enhanced by my latest blood results which were perfect. It had been 10 months since my treatment and, side effects aside, so far so good. On Boxing Day, we wrapped Isla's presents, ready for her party the following day. We were awakened early on her birthday by Geraldine's phone buzzing. She fumbled round in the darkness and got to it just as it stopped. She brought it close to her face – six missed calls from Caroline. She sat up to call her sister back. I lay back, took a deep breath and readied myself for what was to come for her. She was crying within seconds of hearing her sister's voice. I spent the next hour consoling her, making calls and booking flights. By that evening we were back in her family home in Ireland surrounded by relatives and friends. Leo lay in his casket in the front room. I watched with pride as Mary and her two dutiful daughters, with hearts breaking, fussed over the many visitors who flooded their family home. I would occasionally catch Geraldine's bloodshot eyes and ask her if there was anything I could do. I kept asking until I finally worked out my role and found myself a seat in the living room. My only purpose was to be there for her and nothing else. Just to be there for my wife. She'd been there for me so many times – through the loss of my parents, the highs and lows of my career, and the recent loss of my health to heart disease and cancer.

I sat, ignored and ignoring the many well-wishers who streamed through the kitchen, into the living room, then into the front room to view Leo, and back to the kitchen for tea and sandwiches. Mary asked me more than once if I wanted to go in and pay my respects to my dead father-in-law. I politely declined on every occasion. I was worried that my refusal might seem offensive, but it wasn't intended to be. I still carry the scars and memories of seeing my own mother lying dead in a coffin, and that was more than 30 years ago. I vowed then I would never look at another corpse. I haven't since.

Instead of viewing Leo in his casket I stayed rooted in my chair in his living room. I looked up at the family portrait that dominated the wall opposite me. In it, a proud Leo stood tall and grinned widely back at me. By his side was Mary, and in front of him sat his two beautiful daughters. That was his world and he quietly revelled in it. I remembered the day the photo was taken. It was taken in this very room by the wedding photographer who was doing an extra day's work the day after our big day. I was in the room at the time but I'm not in the photo. I was standing to the right of Leo, holding some contraption to enable the photographer to get the best lighting for his masterpiece. Mary and Leo had wanted one last photo of their family before life took them all in different directions. Life did take them in different directions. Geraldine was destined to spend all of her adult life in England with me and her three boys. Caroline went on to marry David and have three girls of her own. But they never stopped being a family. I looked around the living room and back to the photo.

I remembered the first time I'd met Leo. I was a terrified, shy, spotty 15-year-old about to head off to England to pursue a footballing dream. Back then, he can't have thought that he would see much more of me after I left for Newcastle. He was probably relieved I was moving on from his 14-year-old daughter. But I remember how he was with me. He was full of questions and quiet respect. That day we discovered a shared love of music and family that lasted us through 40 years. Forty years where he'd only ever showed me kindness. He'd shown me love and respect above and beyond. In return I loved him. I'm still grateful to him every day for the beautiful young girl who sat in front of him in the portrait on the wall. I raised my glass to the quiet man. To Leo McCaugherty. I thanked him for his life. I thanked him for Geraldine.

CHAPTER 32

If 2018 ended badly, then 2019 started in the same vein. Conor and Kayleigh's relationship ended in early February. I felt a sickness in the pit of my stomach for them both. We'd welcomed Kayleigh into our family, and I know she enjoyed being part of it. I was sad that an important chapter in both their lives was ending. More than that though, my thoughts turned to Isla, now two years old, who had become the centre of our familial universe since her arrival. She was loved and adored by her uncles, Owen and Ciaran, was doted on by Geraldine, and was undoubtedly the best thing that had happened in my life for as long as I could remember. I wanted the world for her, and I still do.

To know that she was now to be part of a broken home, a fractured family, was a gut-wrenching reality I really didn't want for her. She was loved and cared for by all sides of the family, but there was now uncertainty about her future. In the early days of the separation we tried to support Conor and Kayleigh through the turmoil they were in. Geraldine, who has always been more pragmatic than me, was confident they would both do the right thing by Isla and all would fall into place in a 'new normal' for her.

I spent most of my time worrying that we'd somehow lose touch with our only grandchild. I fretted that this bundle of love and joy might be in danger of slipping away from us. I feared that Isla would never truly get to know how much she meant to me, what she meant to all of us. I was terrified that she would somehow miss out on the unconditional love and support we would shower on her.

I needn't have caused myself so much stress. It quickly became apparent that I should have had more faith in the two young people going through the pain of a break-up. They talked together and agreed from the outset that they would continue to raise their daughter as equal parents. They'd make all the big decisions together. Isla would spend half of her time with Kayleigh and half with Conor. The days and weeks that followed were spent converting two rooms in our home. One became a bedroom for Isla and the other was converted into a bedroom and office for Conor. Our home was their home for as long as they needed it. Just when we should have been getting used to an empty house, ours was filled again with the laughter and joy that only a child can bring. We got to spend precious time with Isla that I will always treasure.

By mid-March, the year that had started so badly was taking an enormous turn for the better. Negotiations with potential partners were progressing well and looked like yielding 25 to 50 new Speedflex studios right across the UK, on an 18-month roll-out plan. Isla was happy and content living with us. My latest oncology appointment had been another positive one – my PSA was undetectable again. Apart from some ongoing trouble with muscle soreness and joint pain from my heart medications, all was good again. It was about to get even better.

An email from Guy informed me that he was in advanced negotiations to sell the TV and film rights for *The Boy on the Shed*. He cautioned me not to get too excited, but I paid no attention to him. I danced around the living room until Geraldine came in from the kitchen and embarrassed me into sitting back down and behaving like an adult. After a flurry of further emails over the next week an agreement was reached in principle. Two weeks later I was on my way to BAFTA again, this time to meet Jacqui Miller Charlton and Christian Piers Betley, the transatlantic production team that would be responsible for taking my story to the big screen or TV. Jacqui's home base was Newcastle, while Christian's was Vancouver, though he worked out of Los Angeles. I had a much more relaxed visit to BAFTA than my last frantic effort. We had lunch with Guy and they discussed their plans to take the project forward. I left all three of them talking over lunch as I slipped to the bathroom to change my pad. I washed my hands and stared at the mirror. I allowed myself a wry smile at the absurdity of it all.

The book continued to surpass all expectations I'd had for it. It was still selling well, the reviews were amazing, and it had now won multiple awards. In fact, the only remaining awards ceremony in the industry was The British Sports Book Awards. It was a grand affair that I'd been invited to the year before, held at Lord's Cricket Ground. The great and good of the sporting world were all there. In 2018 I'd attended only as a guest, but this year my invite was as one of the shortlisted authors for Sports Autobiography of the Year. I researched some of the other books on the shortlist and noted the famous names of the authors.

After that particular exercise, I travelled to London more in hope than expectation that my book could possibly win. I was very aware by now that my book was well regarded. The previous awards, the reviews and the film/TV deal told me as much. As with some of the previous awards, I had my doubts that the judges would regard it as a genuine sports book. I hadn't written it as such and had never really believed it was a sports book at all. So I thought it more likely that the judges might favour a big-name sports star's autobiography, which would also guarantee good press coverage for the event itself.

I sat through the long evening next to Guy, Roddy, Karen and Fiona again. My ill-fitting dinner suit dug into my waist and constricted my chest. Awards and winners came and went until finally at the very end of the evening it was time to announce who had won the Sports Autobiography of the Year 2019. The host, former cricketer David Gower, expertly ran through the runners and riders. My suit was getting tighter by the second. I told myself it didn't matter if I didn't win, just being there was a remarkable achievement. But my pounding chest and wet brow were indications that 'I' wasn't listening to 'me'. I wanted to win; I really wanted to win. David brought Catherine Grainger, the great Olympian, on stage to announce the winner. She did. It was me.

It was me! It was *The Boy on the Shed*. I knew I'd won before she announced it. I knew I'd won as soon as she'd said, 'The winner of the Sports Autobiography of the Year is probably the least well-known of the shortlisted contenders.' She was being kind. There was no 'probably' about it. If the award was going to the least well-known author in the room, then it was going to me. I made my way to the stage in a daze and took the trophy from her. I thanked the four cheering people at my table and the two most important women in my life, one of whom was following the event live on Twitter and the other who'd left this world 32 years before. The one following on Twitter had more belief than I had that I would win. The one who'd gone long ago wouldn't have been able to comprehend her son winning any kind of literary prize. But she would have burst with pride at the thought.

A video message of congratulations from Alan Shearer ended my moment in the spotlight and I was whisked off to a quiet room for a quick interview. I made my way back to the main room just as everybody was getting up to leave. I pushed against the tide to reach my table. It was half-deserted.

'Your taxi is outside Paul. Huge congratulations and well deserved.'

Fiona was hugging me as she spoke.

I looked around the room. Five minutes ago I was on the stage enjoying one of the greatest achievements of my life. Now the stage was being dismantled. The night was most definitely over. I shook hands with a couple of stragglers and made my way to the taxi. My phone lit up with messages of congratulations. Geraldine called. She was emotional, and implored me to enjoy the rest of the night. *What rest of the night?* I got back to my hotel at just after 11 p.m., and I made my way to the small bar on the first floor. A middle-aged couple were just finishing their drinks and getting up to leave. There was no one else there. I sat my heavy glass trophy on the table next to the bar. A young man with slicked black hair was leaning over the till. He had his back to me. I cleared my throat and was about to ask him for a glass of wine when he turned and spoke.

'Sorry sir, the bar is closed.'

I looked at my trophy and back at him.

'Is it possible to get a glass of wine to take to my room?'

I guided his eyes to the table where my prize sat proudly perched. He barely glanced at it before emptying a small tray of nuts into the bin below his feet. I picked up my trophy that meant nothing to him and everything to me. I held it against my chest. He was unimpressed and unmoved.

'Congratulations sir, but I'm afraid the bar is still closed.'

With that, he turned his back on me and my trophy. I made my way to my room. My phone continued to buzz with messages of congratulations. I burst out of my suit and changed my pad. Then I searched around the room for something I could drink to celebrate my win. I lay back on my bed and watched *The Simpsons* on TV. I toasted my win with a cup of hot chocolate and a three-pack of Jaffa Cakes, and vowed to learn how to do awards ceremonies better in the future.

* * *

It was late summer 2019. I was driving to my latest oncology appointment, still basking in the glory of *The Boy on the Shed* being voted Sports Autobiography of the Year. I was flicking through the stations and settled on a TalkSPORT interview with Michael Owen. He was promoting his new book. I was interested to hear what he might have to say about his time at Newcastle United. I'd written about my experiences of a short eight-week stint at Newcastle United in 2009, as part of Alan Shearer's management team. In *The Boy on the Shed*, I'd referred to the fact that Michael had injured his groin in the build-up to our penultimate game against Fulham. We'd scanned the injury and whatever it was, it wasn't a serious problem. I'd written how, as a representative of the management team, I'd attended a meeting to discuss Michael's injury and his chances of taking part in our most vital game of the season. Michael was our best chance of scoring the goal against Fulham that might win the game for us, and save the club from relegation. In the presence of the club doctor and the physiotherapists, I'd asked Michael if he felt he would be available for the game. He held his hand over his groin, said he didn't feel too bad, but he was worried that he was out of contract in the summer. He was concerned that if he played and injured himself then he wouldn't get a contract at another club. As part of a management team, I didn't share his reasoning. I reminded him he already had a contract. He had a contract with us. Two days later, on the morning of the Fulham game, he failed a fitness test and didn't play.

Now, 10 years later, I was curious to hear what Michael had to say about his time at the club. Earlier in the month he'd been involved in a Twitter spat with Alan Shearer. He'd already given his version of events during several TV and radio interviews. I liked Michael, but he'd clearly been pricked by what I'd written in my book. I knew he'd been irked, because some friends had drawn my attention to social media comments he'd made after the publication of *The Boy on the Shed*. I hadn't quite realised just how annoyed he was, until I listened to him on the radio that morning. Michael explained how Alan Shearer blamed him for Newcastle's relegation because he thought he hadn't been willing to put his body on the line in the last game of the season against Aston Villa. He then informed his host that he knew why Alan had come to such a conclusion. It was because there was one particular physio there (me) who was 'Alan's go-to man.' I had fed Alan a line about Michael being unwilling to put his body on the line. I was stunned. His recollections of that period were certainly very different to mine. I was frustrated that I didn't have the opportunity to challenge them. So I talked to the radio instead:

'It was the *Fulham* game. Not the *Aston Villa* game. You *were* worried about putting your body on the line. I wasn't a physio or Alan's "go-to" man. I was part of his management team. Your management team. You were our captain.'

When he'd finished his interview and I had finished talking to the radio, I realised I'd pulled the car over to the side of the road. I was frustrated that nothing he'd said had been questioned or fact-checked. One simple question about the Fulham game and not the Aston Villa game would have sufficed to contradict everything that he'd just presented. I thought about phoning the station. I felt entitled to, as he'd just made a direct reference to me and my book. He'd done so while delivering a version of events I simply didn't recognise. Then I looked at the clock, and realised I was going to be late for my oncology appointment. I shook my head and smiled. What was coming out of the radio really no longer mattered that much. I had bigger concerns to deal with today. I swapped the interview for Spotify. *Madame George* changed my mood. Van Morrison took me all the way to the Freeman Hospital. I was grateful he still mattered to me.

Dr Frew was happy with my progress. So much so, that I was now only required to go through the nervous ordeal of checking my bloods every six months instead of every three. A small victory, but a victory all the same. I could forget about my prostate cancer for a few months. Instead, I could concentrate on my work, my family and my writing. I could also focus on trying to sort out the constant muscle and joint pain that had plagued me for three or four years since my heart attack. I'd initially been convinced the cause was my statin medication. I was sure it was my statins that had me feeling 20 years older than I was. Yet, no matter how many times I'd adjusted them or stopped taking them altogether, my aches and pains were still with me to varying degrees. I think my GP was becoming as baffled as me as to why that was, and I was still dealing with the side effects of my cancer treatment. They were challenges, no doubt.

Regardless, I had several reasons to be positive. My bloods were good. We were making real progress with Speedflex. I had written another manuscript and was halfway through writing this one. My regular conversations with Christian had culminated in him travelling from Vancouver just before Christmas 2019. He spent a few days with me in Newcastle and in Ireland, identifying locations for the filming of *The Boy on the Shed*.

The new year fizzed into life full of brilliant promise. We opened three Speedflex studios in London and hosted an event with industry insiders at one of those locations. It bore great fruit. At dinner afterwards, I received commitments from huge players in the fitness industry. We were on our way. In early February, I had an exciting lunch with the scriptwriter/director and producers who were adapting my novel, *An Irish Heartbeat,* into a feature film. My diary was full with work and my spare time was filled with Isla and my writing. A whole new avenue was also opening up for me. Following the success of *The Boy on the Shed*, I was now receiving regular requests for public speaking engagements. I was loving every minute of them. Then the whole world stopped. It was 23 March 2020.

CHAPTER 33

Like everyone else, I watched as the COVID-19 pandemic swept across the world. Images from China, and Italy, had given us all plenty of warning of what was to come. But what was to come was worse than anyone could ever have imagined. As the UK death toll rose, everything ground to a shuddering halt. I was 'furloughed', became part of a 'support bubble', and was identified as 'clinically vulnerable' long before I really understood what these new words and phrases actually meant.

I spent the first few days of the March 2020 lockdown reassuring our young staff at Speedflex they would all receive their salaries in full. I was grateful to Graham Wylie, who had agreed to foot the bill. Geraldine was sent home from her teaching job at school and some unresolved blood pressure issues meant she, too, was confined to our home. In the following weeks and months we adapted to our alternative reality. We hid from the world and made sure we did all we could to stay safe. As weeks bled into months, the life we had previously known simply vanished. But our lives didn't just stop. Like everyone else, we had to find new ways to *be*.

Family life moved on. Owen caught the virus in the first wave. Luckily, he was living away from home at the time so we were protected from it. Unluckily for him, it really affected his breathing and it was touch and go at one point as to whether he needed to pay a visit to the local hospital. Thankfully, at 23 years old, and fit and healthy, he avoided the need for that intervention. He came back home to live in the summer. He was then imprisoned here, during the next lockdown. He worked and slept in his bedroom, unable to go anywhere or do anything until the restrictions were lifted. His social life disappeared and eventually his job did too. Always easy-going, the pandemic has forced him to re-evaluate what and where he wants to be in life. It turned his world upside down. He is still trying to find his way through the fallout. I'm confident he will. Ciaran was trapped here during the first lockdown. He got caught up in the national scandal that was the A-level algorithm fiasco. His predicted grades were all downgraded by the computer. He suffered the crushing experience of being awarded grades well below anything he had achieved in his entire lifetime at school. Thankfully, the error was corrected, and he headed off to university in September 2020 to study law and catch COVID himself. At 19, it barely laid a glove on him. After a year of online lectures and closed pubs, he has finally been able to enjoy student life as it is meant to be. Conor's music management career ground to a standstill overnight. He had 60 gigs cancelled in one day. He and his new partner Amy were forced apart by the restrictions, but this seemed only to strengthen their bond. In the middle of all the chaos, they managed to buy their first home together. It was quite an achievement in the circumstances. Amy has bonded with Isla. Their growing love and respect for each other is obvious and heart-warming to see. Geraldine's hip replacement surgery vanished over the horizon. She was in constant and severe pain. It was more than sad to witness my previously active wife struggle to lift herself from the chair before she hobbled her way around the house. Her blood pressure issues were resolved. This meant that by the commencement of the second lockdown she was back to limping her way around school instead of home. But not before we'd spent our spring and summer creating endless adventures with Isla.

Our three-year-old granddaughter was the sunshine in our family. She kept us all going through the long weeks and months. We were worried at first how we were going to keep her occupied when everything and everywhere was closed. We shouldn't have fretted. In the early days of April we discovered the forest on our doorstep. What I'd previously assumed was just a line of trees bordering the farmland next to our home turned out to be a stunning forest playground for

Isla, and for all of us. We'd just never taken the time to really explore our surroundings before. Our daily walk in the forest became an endless adventure when observed through the eyes of a child who saw magic everywhere. We searched for fairy houses, splashed in the stream, found a secret island, played hide and seek, and marvelled at the deer who often walked across our path. We shouted to the trees and listened for our voices to call back to us. We didn't just leave the magic in the forest – we brought it back home with us, too. Every day she visited us she would rush into the living room. She would search everywhere until she found what she was looking for. She'd then check to see if there was any magic in her magic tin. Every single time she would find some new magic. Inside her tin, without fail, there would always be a little gift – a small toy or some sweets. The tin itself was nothing special. It was small and round and it had once been home to three tubs of Vaseline, but to Isla, it was magic. Every evening she'd make sure her tin was open. Only if it was open could the magic find its way in.

We were walking in the forest in early autumn. She was holding my hand. Conor was walking behind us.

'Who puts the magic in my magic tin?'

She had suddenly stopped and tugged my hand. I turned to face her. She beckoned me closer so her daddy couldn't hear her doubting the magic. I smiled at her.

'I don't know. It's just magic. Who do you think puts the magic in the tin?'

She raised her palms, tilted her head, and then pointed at me.

'I think it's you granda. I think you put the magic in the tin. Don't you?'

I leaned down so her face was nearly touching mine. I lied to her.

'If it was me, then surely I'd know what was in it when you open it? But every time you open it, you have to tell me what's inside. So it can't be me. It must just be magic.'

She smiled back at me.

'So it *is* magic. Like the fairies and the reindeers and the echoes?'

I looked into her wide eyes and lied to her again.

'It is magic.'

We stood for a moment looking at each other. She was content. The tin was magic after all.

* * *

When Geraldine returned to teaching, and Isla started nursery, the inevitable happened and COVID found its way into our previously impenetrable home. Isla and Conor brushed it off but for me and Geraldine it resulted in a worrying and debilitating couple of weeks. Neither of us were ever in any real danger as it turned out, but the fear of not knowing where this virus could take either of us was almost as bad as any physical discomfort we endured. I was so worried about ending up in hospital that I religiously followed some breathing exercises and forced coughing. I'd watched a very helpful doctor demonstrate them on video and diligently practised the recommended technique four times a day. I did it so much that by the end of the two weeks I had a lump protruding from my abdomen just above the scar where my prostate had been removed. I'd coughed my way to a hernia. Geraldine fully recovered from COVID and I've been left with a mild reduction in my ability to differentiate tastes and smells. I now regularly smell smoke and find myself searching around for non-existent fires. We fared better than so many who were less fortunate than us.

* * *

It's December 2021. Life hasn't fully returned to what it was before COVID. But it's getting there. The infection rates are high. While the vaccines have saved many lives, there are still too many people dying. It feels like we are moving out of the worst of it, but the threat of new variants remains. Geraldine had her hip replaced in February. Her pain has gone but her other hip is starting to creak. I know it's frustrating for her, but she never complains. She is her usual upbeat self and takes everything this life throws at her with calm fortitude. I wish I was more like her. I'm proud that someone like her chose someone like me to share her good times and bad. I've given her more bad times than good in recent years. My failing health looms large over us. I am in a battle. I know that I am. I've had some victories. I am no longer incontinent. The early signs are that the injection therapy will work for me. Most importantly, my PSA is undetectable nearly four years after my radiotherapy. I get it tested every six months.

I am still in a fight. I have heart disease and I have prostate cancer. My two opponents would be hard to beat individually but together they make it an unfair contest. Two versus one is never a fair fight. They pack quite a punch. Ultimately, one might knock me out before my time is up, but I am determined to take them the distance. The lockdowns have given me too much time to think with not enough of life's distractions to occupy my restless mind. I am broken. Of that there is no doubt. Physically, a part of me is missing and it's never coming back. I am not the man I once was. Mentally, I have yet to come to terms with the man I have become. The boy on the shed has become the man on the ledge. Clinging on and gripping tight to stop myself from falling.

The night-times are the worst. My formidable opponents hit hardest in the loneliness of the darkness. They wake me from my sleep and their onslaught is relentless. They torture me with my own fears. As they rain their blows down on me, I hold on to Geraldine while she sleeps, just to feel she is there. They hit me with one low blow after another.

I won't be there to share Geraldine's old age. I'll cause her unnecessary hardship. I won't see my children's families grow. I won't be around long enough for my precious granddaughter to remember who I was. She'll know nothing of the unconditional love and kindness I showered on her, the games we played together or the adventures we had. I will be an old photograph that my children show theirs. I'll be nothing but a half-told story at some drunken family get-together.

I cling on. I take their blows until sleep rings its bell and gives me respite until morning. They are still with me when I awake but their punches lack the power of the night before. I pull on my training kit and search for my trainers while they whisper in my ear:

*Have a cup of tea. It's freezing outside. You will slip and fall. Train
tomorrow instead. Haven't you got some urgent emails to send? Your
knee is a bit sore; you'll only make it worse.*

I ignore them. I open the door and drag them with me into the
lane. I start running. With every step I punch them back. They are on
the ropes now. I get to the junction half a mile from the house and
they are counterpunching.

*Go left, down the hill. It's the easiest route. It will be kinder on your
knee.*

I go right. Every time. I run up the winding hill. When I get near
the top and I'm almost spent, I run harder and I run faster, until my
legs are burning, and I can feel my heart bursting out of my chest. My
opponents fall silent when I reach the summit, beaten to a pulp. But
this morning they hit me with an unexpected sucker punch.

I was gulping in the winter air, admiring the clear blue sky that
capped the picture-perfect landscape below. I took my first step to
head back down the hill but lost my footing. I slipped on some black
ice. I tried to steady myself with my other foot but it slid, too. I started
to windmill my legs, in a desperate attempt to stop my fall, but my
whirling legs left the ground in unison. I hovered in the air for a
brief moment. Then I crashed down to earth. My back took the first
blow and then my head followed. I lay there on the hill. An icy river
made its way down the inside of my top. It flowed unimpeded into
my bottoms and found a resting place in my training shoes. Every
part of me hurt as I lay there on that freezing hill. My opponents
had knocked me down. I lay there defeated. A tear left my eye and
made its way into my ear. It shocked me that I was crying. Then I
realised I wasn't. It wasn't sadness I was feeling. It wasn't defeat. It was
anger. It was raw, powerful anger that I had to forever carry these two
destructive bastards around with me. I cursed my heart disease and
the side effects of the medication. I cursed my prostate cancer that
had stolen away the man I used to be. I looked up at the blue sky and I
swore at the universe beyond it. When I was done, I got up. I checked
the cuts on my head and my hand. I made sure my knee was able to
support my weight. Then I began to hobble. I began to walk. I started

to run. And run. And run. I ran all the way home. I *am* in a fight. A fight for my life. But I am up for that fight.

It's late afternoon now and I'm on my way to pick up Isla. On the wall opposite where I'm typing these words hangs my favourite Christmas present from December 2020. It is a framed photograph, taken in early autumn in the forest. It is of Isla and me at that very moment when she was asking me who put the magic in her tin. Conor captured us in mid-conversation. We are leaning into each other and smiling. The sun is as harsh on my face as it is kind on hers. The past and the future together forever. It was a moment I knew at the time I would treasure. I still don't know why. I know that she will spend most of her journey on this planet without my presence in her life. That is a sad fact. But we are both here now. That is enough. I am part of her and she is part of me. If, when she is older, hopefully much older, someone should ask about her granda, I hope she smiles and thinks of love, kindness, adventures and magic. And that reminds me. I have one more job to do before I leave to pick her up. I go to the drawer in the kitchen and take out the contents. I make my way to the living room. I pick up the old tin that is sitting open on the couch. I slip the contents into it and close the lid. I haven't put any magic in there, just the contents for her to find later. The magic doesn't happen until Isla sees it there. I didn't lie to her in the forest. It isn't me. It's her. Isla, my four-year-old granddaughter. She chooses to see the magic in the tin.

I get it now. My heart attack and my cancer diagnosis so soon afterwards were punishing blows to take. They rocked me off my feet. But my heart attack didn't kill me and my cancer hasn't either. They are merely unwelcome intruders who have prevented me from seeing the magic I once saw all around me in this life. I've been too frightened to look for it again. I was scared that it might be gone forever.

I look at the photo again like I'm looking at it for the first time. I see now why I treasured the moment. It's staring me right in the face. She is looking at me through my mother's eyes. She has my mother's eyes. There is magic in that. I glance at the old tin nestling on the chair. It looks different to me now than it did just moments ago. I make my way to the door. Snow is falling. Autumn has gone and winter is here. But there is magic to be found in winter too. I close the door behind me. I look up and breathe in the cold air. The snow caresses my face. It feels just like it did when I was a child. I'm ready now. I'm ready for the magic.

I'm ready to see the magic in the tin.

ACKNOWLEDGMENTS

I would like to thank my wife Geraldine for her unwavering love and support, and her endless patience while having to read and re-read the manuscript. I must also thank Kerry McDonnell, my other unofficial proofreader for her encouraging feedback. Thank you to Alan Shearer for his enduring friendship and (yet another) foreword. Thanks also to Michael Walker for his support. To my agent Guy Rose, a sincere thank you once again for ensuring my words found a great home. I feel an enormous sense of gratitude towards my editor Matt Lowing who has shown unflinching belief in my story from the very beginning. It has been a pleasure to be guided through this process by him. A heartfelt thank you to Zoë Blanc, whose insightful edits and hard work have ensured my words are presented in the best possible light. I must also thank Katherine Macpherson for ensuring the book reaches as wide a readership as possible. I would like to acknowledge my boys, Conor, Owen, and Ciaran, who have enriched my life more than they will ever know. Once they get over the embarrassment of some of the content in the book, I hope they will take pride in the courage it took to write it. I want to mention Stanley Dewart. Thanks for the friendship and the many lifts to the airport on cold winter mornings a lifetime ago, Stan. My final thank you is to my granddaughter Isla. This book would never have been written without the inspiration she provided.

It was written for you, Isla.

Love,
Granda x